Therapeutic Pluralism

The profile of complementary and alternative medicine (CAM) has risen dramatically over the last decade and cancer patients represent its most prolific users. As a result, the NHS and UK cancer services are attempting to develop a wider range of therapeutic options for patients. Despite such developments, little is known about why cancer patients use CAM, its perceived benefits and the perspectives of the doctors and nurses involved.

Drawing on extensive fieldwork in the UK, *Therapeutic Pluralism* includes over 120 interviews with cancer patients and professionals, plus innovative 'diary' data which, for the first time, detail the experiences of CAM users. It gives a systematic analysis of issues such as:

- the development of patient preferences and influences on decision-making;
- expectations of CAM and interpretations of 'success' in cancer treatment;
- the nature and importance of 'evidence' and 'effectiveness' for patients;
- the organisational dynamics involved in integrating CAM into the NHS;
- pathways to CAM and the role of the Internet;
- the role of oncology clinicians in patients' experiences of cancer and their use of CAMs.

Therapeutic Pluralism is essential reading for students and researchers of medical sociology, complementary and alternative medicine, and cancer. It will also be useful to medical and health professionals, and policymakers with an interest in complementary and alternative medicine.

Alex Broom is a Lecturer in Sociology at the University of Newcastle, Australia.

Philip Tovey is a Reader in Health Sociology at the School of Healthcare, University of Leeds, United Kingdom.

Therapeutic Pluralism

Exploring the experiences of cancer patients and professionals

Alex Broom and Philip Tovey

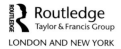

Routledge
Taylor & Francis Group

LONDON AND NEW YORK

First published 2008
by Routledge
2 Park Square, Milton Park, Abingdon, Oxon OX14 4RN

Simultaneously published in the USA and Canada
by Routledge
270 Madison Ave., New York, NY 10016

Routledge is an imprint of the Taylor & Francis Group, an informa business

Typeset in Times New Roman by
RefineCatch Limited, Bungay, Suffolk
Printed and bound in Great Britain by
TJ International Ltd, Padstow, Cornwall

British Library Cataloguing in Publication Data
A catalogue record for this book is available from the British Library

Library of Congress Cataloging in Publication Data
Broom, Akex.
   Therapeutic pluralism : exploring the experiences of cancer patients
and professionals / Alex Broom & Philip Tovey.
      p. ; cm.
   Includes bibliographical references and index.
   1. Cancer—Alternative treatment—Great Britain.   I. Tovey, Philip,
1963–   II. Title. [DNLM: 1. Neoplasms—therapy.
2. Complementary Therapies—methods. QZ 266 B873t 2008]
   RC271.A62B73 2008
   616.99′406—dc22

                                                                2007034039

ISBN 10: 0-415-39852-5 (hbk)
ISBN 10: 0-415-39853-3 (pbk)
ISBN 10: 0-203-89445-6 (ebk)

ISBN 13: 978-0-415-39852-7 (hbk)
ISBN 13: 978-0-415-39853-4 (pbk)
ISBN 13: 978-0-203-89445-3 (ebk)

For
Lucy, Jen and Sarah
Georgia – still gorgeous, now peachy

Contents

**2 The role of the Internet in cancer patients' engagement with
therapeutic options**

**3 Integrating CAM: a comparative analysis of hospice versus
hospital medicine**

**4 Oncologists' and specialist cancer nurses' approaches to CAM
and their impact on patient action**

Acknowledgements

First, we want to thank the patients and the clinicians who kindly gave their time to share their experiences with us. Without their willingness to tell their stories this book would not have been possible. Thanks also to members of the original project team, including Marianne Tavares, Mike Stockton, Dawn Alison and Francine Cheater. We would also like to thank the Department of Health for funding this project. Parts of Chapter 3 originally appeared in the *Sociology of Health and Illness*, vol. 29, no. 3. Parts of Chapter 4 originally appeared in *Social Science and Medicine*, vol. 64, no. 12. Parts of Chapter 1 originally appeared in *Sociology* vol. 41, no. 6.

Abbreviations

BMA	British Medical Association
CAM	Complementary and alternative medicine
CRUK	Cancer Research United Kingdom
DoH	Department of Health
EBCAM	Evidence-based complementary and alternative medicine
EBM	Evidence-based medicine
EBP	Evidence-based practice
GP	General practitioner
NHS	National Health Service
NICE	National Institute for Health and Clinical Excellence
PCT	Primary Care Trust
RCCM	Research Council for Complementary Medicine
RCP	The Royal College of Physicians
RCT	Randomised controlled trial
TCM	Traditional Chinese Medicine
UK	United Kingdom

Introduction

Complementary and alternative medicine (CAM) has become a high-profile issue in the last two decades, and in the context of cancer care it is both prominent and controversial. Use of CAM by cancer patients in the United Kingdom (UK) is considerable and calls for increased public provision are frequent. Research continues to illustrate high levels of individual patient usage (e.g. Ernst and Cassileth, 1998; Fouladbakhsh *et al.*, 2005; Lewith *et al.*, 2002; Rees *et al.*, 2000; J. Scott *et al.*, 2005) and there exists a substantial divide between public preference for therapeutic alternatives and National Health Service (NHS) provision. CAM, at least in a limited form, is now considered a fairly standard element of palliative care in the UK, with a recent report emphasising the integral nature of CAM to end-of-life care (Tavares, 2003). Whilst broad shifts towards integration have been evident in the treatment of more advanced disease, hospital-based cancer services have shown less propensity to accept non-biomedical options and, as such, are coming under increased political and public pressure to move beyond a *purely* biomedical-type service provision (Broom and Tovey, 2007). However, despite considerable advocacy on the part of political lobby groups, grassroots patient support networks and the volunteer sector, hospital-based oncology services currently provide very little in the way of non-biomedical therapeutics, and even in palliative care contexts CAM services are limited in scope and lack formalised financial backing from the NHS.

The issue of CAM integration in cancer care has also been played out in the political arena in the last decade. The high-profile House of Lords report in 2000 called for increased research on the issue of CAM (House of Lords, 2000) and emphasised the need for greater momentum in the movement toward a more integrative (but also evidence-based) form of patient care. Moreover, national cancer policy now espouses a more rounded (and less solely medical) approach (Department of Health, 2000, 2004) and CAM and cancer is high on the Department of Health's (DoH) agenda.

Regardless of considerable public support and the increasingly political nature of the issue, in practice UK cancer care is still largely biomedical in emphasis. Thus, despite an increasingly pluralistic public sphere and increased political rhetorical around 'integration', at the point of service delivery treatment remains firmly ideologically positioned around the biomedical model and monolithic in approach to patient care. There are, however, very small (but significant) pockets of integration that are now emerging in the UK, with *some* NHS-supported hospices and hospital-based cancer services providing limited CAM services to cancer patients.

Such developments have been driven by a powerful UK volunteer sector, focused on providing cancer patients with therapeutic alternatives outside the mainstream, as well as bolstering existing NHS-provided supportive cancer care facilities. This has led to some NHS Trusts, albeit with considerable scepticism, accepting on-site CAM services, with volunteer-funded centres operating within cancer facilities and providing therapies not funded (nor explicitly condoned) by the NHS, the DoH or the National Institute for Clinical Excellence (NICE) (see Broom and Tovey, 2007). Ideologically, such developments have the potential to fundamentally alter the nature of cancer care as 'non-evidence-based' CAMs are included in a previously biomedically dominated landscape. In practice, and as examined in the following chapters, the UK cancer services (including their practitioners, policies, organisational structures, funding rules and strategies of community engagement) are reacting and evolving in subtle but important ways in an attempt to manage the range of issues presented by the increasing interplay between CAM and biomedicine. This is producing a subtle but important process of organisationally specific strategic evolution that has considerable implications for the nature of biomedicine, CAM and cancer care in the United Kingdom and internationally.

This book provides a sociologically informed examination of the impacts of, and responses to, CAM in the UK cancer services. Within our analysis presented in the following chapters we examine the impact of the interplay between CAM and biomedicine for individuals (i.e. patients and practitioners), organisations (i.e. NHS Trusts and the hospice movement), ideologies (i.e. integrative care/the biomedical model) and current trajectories in healthcare delivery (i.e. evidence-based medicine and evidence-based practice). What results is a critical exploration into how CAM is reconfiguring individual experience of disease, grassroots professional practice, inter-professional dynamics and NHS organisational culture. Departing from the traditional focus on simplistic (and positivist) notions of clinical effectiveness and treatment efficacy, here we examine how these very ideas about legitimacy are constructed, deployed, contested and reconfigured by differently positioned social actors (including patients, doctors, nurses and CAM therapists). As a result of the arguments presented in the following chapters we argue that for progress to be made in cancer care, and before CAM 'integration' is even considered as a policy trajectory, we must *first* explore and unravel the complex ideological, territorial and epistemological issues evident at the intersections of (and conflicts between) CAM and biomedicine.

Empirical, theoretical and historical context

In order to embark on a critical sociological examination of CAM in cancer care, it is useful to first provide an overview of the key issues that have been debated in the medical and sociological literature, such as: defining 'complementary' or 'alternative' medicine; patterns in CAM consumption within the population; the character of cancer care in the UK; sites of inequality in cancer care and CAM consumption; and cancer clinicians' views of CAM. Thus, in the following discussion we provide an overview of existing literature exploring these key areas, followed by a critical overview of the theoretical ideas in sociology that have been applied to CAM. As such, this chapter provides a substantive and theoretical platform that informs the analysis presented in the following chapters.

What is CAM?

A key question in the sociological literature in the context of CAM has been: what constitutes a complementary or alternative medicine? Indeed, we have seen an evolution in terminology over the last decade, including such labels as 'alternative', 'natural', 'folk', 'holistic', 'unproven' and 'complementary'. Each is ideologically loaded in its own unique way and, importantly, each has presented significant difficulties to both CAM and biomedical practitioners. Ultimately, such terminology has become problematic because each category caries with it assumptions about the character of CAM, effectiveness and rigour, as well as potential therapeutic benefits (see Broom, 2002). Each category holds certain qualities that neither CAM practitioners nor biomedical practitioners have (unanimously) accepted. *Complementary*, as a category, is for many CAM practitioners to be considered 'non-essential'. *Alternative* is equally problematic, suggesting, for some practitioners, a degree of separation and paradigmatic incommensurability. Moreover, 'alternative', for some biomedical clinicians, denotes legitimacy, in being considered an 'alternative' to biomedical cancer care. Lastly, *unproven* suggests, for CAM therapists, that what distinguishes CAM and biomedical is 'evidence' or 'efficacy'. However, as has been examined in the sociological literature, what constitutes 'evidence' is a hotly disputed topic (Broom and Tovey, 2007). As a result there is still ongoing debate over what CAM *is*, what characterises CAM practices and thus what to call them (e.g. Broom, 2002).

We take a different approach to terminology, in that what interests us here is the impact and durability of certain categories (i.e. natural, holistic or invasive), and, furthermore, the deployment of certain discourses and rhetorical practices (i.e. evidence based, unproven or integrative) through 'commonsense' terminology. Our approach is that CAM is ultimately a constructed and dynamic entity that is historically and culturally variable. Moreover, it contains concrete or 'harder' elements (i.e. basic artefacts such as acupuncture needles or crystals) and softer elements (i.e. ideology, hand movements or approaches to the therapeutic relationship) which are represented in certain ways and categorised as certain things. CAM does not exist *per se*; it has no identifiable, concrete boundaries or borders outside the sense-making practices that we all embark on (including CAM sociologists). Rather, it is a somewhat clumsy (but nevertheless useful) meta-category that helps us impose meanings on practices that are hugely diverse and often paradigmatically disparate.

A key problem for some – and a fascinating feature for us sociologists – is that they (i.e. CAM practices, artefacts, knowledges, institutions, etc.) do not stay still. Rather, actors reposition themselves, they enlist other actors (and artefacts) and they shift, maintaining certain features and drawing in others (see also Broom, 2002). At various points in time there have been *attempts* to establish a lasting definition of CAM; a durable list of which modalities are essentially CAM or biomedicine. As could be predicted, such a list invariably fails the test of time, in that what is CAM is variable over time and space.

This 'problem' of definition/categorisation, and the socially and culturally mobile nature of non-biomedical therapeutics, plagues baseline survey research on CAM. As highlighted by Zollman and Vickers (1999), there is a lack of consistency in definitions of CAM between studies. For example, the inclusion of spiritual practices (which can be anything from praying for healing to consulting a spiritual healer) as CAM greatly increases the percentage of CAM users (see Richardson *et al.*, 2000). Moreover, a flat percentage of 'CAM users' provides little information regarding the usage of particular modalities (i.e. chiropractic versus psychic surgery). Thus, statistics tend to tell us little about which alternative modalities are most frequently used and tend to promote an image of the ascendance of all CAMs, an image that may in fact be inaccurate.

Whilst for some the shifting nature of CAM may represent something of a frustration, for us it represents a key focus of investigation; a reflection of the need for in-depth examination of grassroots processes and evolving communities of practice as CAM becomes increasingly integrated (at least within the public sphere) into contemporary cancer care. Whilst acknowledging the complexities outlined above, a purely constructivist approach provides too little in terms of lines of reference and points of (socially derived) therapeutic delineation. As such, there are some observations we can make about what CAM is at this point of time and in this socio-cultural context.

Broadly, the category 'CAM' is used to refer to a wide range of therapeutic practices, including: aromatherapy, naturopathy, herbalism, homeopathy, reiki, acupuncture, spiritual healing, etc. Moreover, there are certain parallels we can draw between CAMs. What largely characterises CAMs is, first, a lack of integration into Western healthcare systems and, second, their tendency to espouse models of care that incorporate physical and metaphysical elements in treatment processes. There is also some merit in distinguishing between 'whole-systems' approaches like naturopathy or homeopathy and the less ideologically driven healing approaches such as reiki, aromatherapy massage or healing touch. Whilst these categories are disputed and should not be viewed as in any way static, Table 1, from the National Centre for Complementary and Alternative Medicine in the US, provides one (albeit limited) schema for differentiating between different CAMs.

There are similar issues with what to call what many people refer to as 'Western' or 'modern' medicine. Historically, Western medicine (insofar as this is even a valid category in itself) has been referred to as 'modern', 'conventional' or even 'traditional'. However, these categories have obvious limitations. For example, some biomedical techniques and practices developed from what we may consider pre-modern times and, indeed, 'traditional', as a

Table 1 Categories of CAM

Alternative medical systems	Alternative medical systems are built upon complete systems of theory and practice. Often, these systems have evolved apart from and earlier than the conventional medical approach used in the United States. Examples of alternative medical systems that have developed in Western cultures include homeopathic medicine and naturopathic medicine. Examples of systems that have developed in non-Western cultures include Traditional Chinese Medicine and Ayurveda.
Mind–body interventions	Mind–body medicine uses a variety of techniques designed to enhance the mind's capacity to affect bodily function and symptoms, including meditation, prayer, mental healing and therapies that use creative outlets such as art, music or dance.
Biologically based therapies	Biologically based therapies in CAM use substances found in nature, such as herbs, foods and vitamins. Some examples include dietary supplements, herbal products and the use of other so-called natural therapies (for example using shark cartilage to treat cancer).
Manipulative and body-based methods	Manipulative and body-based methods in CAM are based on manipulation and/or movement of one or more parts of the body. Some examples include chiropractic or osteopathic manipulation, and massage.
Energy therapies	Energy therapies involve the use of energy fields. They are of two types: 1 Biofield therapies are intended to affect energy fields that purportedly surround and penetrate the human body. The existence of such fields has not yet been scientifically proven. Some forms of energy therapy manipulate biofields by applying pressure and/or manipulating the body by placing the hands in, or through, these fields. Examples include qi gong, Reiki and Therapeutic Touch. 2 Bioelectromagnetic-based therapies involve the unconventional use of electromagnetic fields, such as pulsed fields, magnetic fields or alternating-current or direct-current fields.

therapeutic category, tends now to denote indigenous medicines in developing countries (see Tovey *et al.*, 2007). Thus, within the following chapters we generally refer to 'Western medicine' as biomedicine. Biomedicine, we argue, is a less loaded term in that it merely refers to the ideological basis of the practices we generally recognise as 'modern' medicine (i.e. techniques based on the application of the principles of the natural sciences and especially biology and biochemistry), rather than suggesting its progressiveness (i.e. modern) or geographical roots (i.e. Western). But a key question in order to understand the current contemporary therapeutic landscape is how biomedicine came to be.

Biomedicine in social context

Western medicine, or *biomedicine* as we will call it here, came into being through a relatively recent process of securing state validation, professional autonomy and self-regulation. Through the implementation of various policies, acts, regulations and laws, biomedicine, in large part, ensured that certain practices did not receive state legitimation (see Willis, 1994). Biomedicine is, ultimately, the product of historical struggles over access to resources, rights to practise, state validation and occupational territories. Throughout these struggles, biomedicine has been relatively successful in establishing a monopoly over the delivery of primary and secondary healthcare. As such, the dominance of biomedicine has been as much about political manoeuvring, and achieving self-regulation, as it has been about effectiveness. Of course, one cannot separate *effectiveness* from access to resources. Alliances, state funding and the flow-on effect of political power all contribute to claims about the legitimacy of the order of things (the dominance of the biomedical model), with resources spent on furthering the biomedical approach, thus boosting the performance of biomedicine over other therapeutic modalities.

Some specific historical knowledge of the evolution of medicine(s) is useful at this point. Just as CAM should be viewed as an evolving and culturally located entity, so too should biomedicine. Whilst the historical dominance of biomedicine (as least in the second half of the twentieth century) has made it seem common sense (as a model of health), and somewhat harder as a sociocultural phenomena (or more immutable), it is nevertheless a relatively recent entity/institution. In Europe, before the widespread emergence of the medical profession, a range of modalities were available, including astrology, herbalism and healing (Larner, 1992). The pattern until the nineteenth century was for different modalities to wax and wane in popularity. However, in the mid-nineteenth century one of these modalities, allopathy (what has now evolved into what we call biomedicine), began to rise into a position of dominance (Willis, 1994). The initial development of the medical profession in England in the nineteenth century came about through the merging of apothecaries, surgeons and physicians (Abbott, 1988). In 1815, the General Pharmaceutical Association initiated the Apothecaries Act, looking to the government to raise the standard of entry into the profession and to prohibit 'unqualified persons' from practising. The Act was the outcome of an ongoing struggle to create defined occupational boundaries between the apothecaries, druggists and chemists, physicians and surgeons (Dew, 1998). This Act introduced the concept of a qualified or registered practitioner into English law, which gave the General Medical Council powers to control who could practise medicine (Waddington, 1973). The 1858 Act was an outright victory for the 'regular' medical practitioners of the day. These political and regulatory struggles fundamentally shaped what we now receive today.

With the dominance of biomedicine came a specific set of understandings about the body, the nature of disease and the patient/provider relationship; what we generally refer to as the *biomedical model*. This model of therapeutic practice espoused ideas that would dramatically alter the treatment of illness and disease in the twentieth and twenty-first centuries. Importantly for this book, these biomedical assumptions and now entrenched treatment practices are crucially relevant to the reasons why patients may utilise CAM, their experiences of biomedical care, and paradigmatic conflict between CAM and biomedicine. As summarised in Table 2, the biomedical model of disease is underpinned by important implicit assumptions such as a dualistic split between the mind and the body, the importance of 'cure' versus healing and the objectivity and thus authority of the expert (see Samson, 1999), all of which are crucial to understanding the implications of the rise of CAM in contemporary therapeutic culture.

The biomedical model, as seen in Table 2, and the embodiment of its assumptions within technological advances are self-perpetuating. If it is accepted that disease is reducible to the organ and cellular levels, then more is spent on technologies which are able to isolate and fix these organ- and cell-specific problems. In doing so, there is an increasingly limited ability to treat disease as anything other than an organ-specific and cellular malfunction as technologies are built to reduce disease reality to these levels. Thus, medical technologies, interventions, practices and policies are intimately involved in the immutability of particular ways of making sense of illness – they capture, define and thus reproduce disease. They are involved in treating, and thus in rendering some things treatable and others untreatable. The result is an

Table 2 The biomedical model

Mechanistic	The body is compartmentalised
Symptomatic	A condition is reduced to a category, a single disease entity, which exhibits a distinctive set of symptoms
Objectivity	The practitioner is separate and detached from the patient, maintaining objectivity, assisted by scientific evidence
Quantification	Information is derived from what can be quantified
Determinism	Phenomena can be predicted from knowledge of scientific laws

increasing reliance on the ability of biomedical experts to discover new and better ways of fixing us – that is, to produce new technologies that can discover (diagnosis), predict (prognosis) and cure – in accordance with the tenets of the biomedical approach.

This mechanistic approach also stresses the central role of the clinician in the healing process. The clinician's intervention is active, and, in general, downplays the role of any mental and emotional factors that may cause the disease or play a role in its natural evolution or treatment. The biomedical model is characterised as materialist in its focus on the corporeal body, yet at the same time abstract in its removal of the body from the soul and from the person. It is important at this point to stress that this is a *model* of healthcare prominent within biomedicine, not a description of the approach generally taken by biomedical practitioners. However, in saying this, the centrality of this model in biomedicine does strongly influence how medical practitioners approach treatment processes.

Importantly for this book, the biomedical view of disease as mechanistic malfunction and of the medical practitioner as the expert repairer still dominates public-health provision, and particularly cancer care, in the UK (B.S. Turner and Samson, 1995). However, this model of care is being increasingly challenged as new therapeutic models compete for legitimacy in a more pluralistic contemporary therapeutic environment. Furthermore, and as reflected in the statistics presented in the next section, the failure of biomedicine to cure (or even decrease the prevalence of) many common cancers has led to a reduction in public deference to biomedical expertise and increased support for CAM therapeutics. The landscape of cancer in the UK is critical here to provide a context for the analysis presented in the following chapters.

Cancer in the United Kingdom

Whilst wider debates about CAM are relevant to the analysis presented in this book, cancer represents a unique and highly emotionally charged disease context within which to explore therapeutic experience. As such, an understanding of the specific character of cancer in the UK and the NHS cancer service is critical to understanding the analysis presented in the following chapters. Whilst broad standards of care do not differ *hugely* across Western industrialised countries like the UK, Canada and Australia, there are certain features of cancer in the UK that warrant attention.

Each year in the UK around 275,000 people are diagnosed with cancer and the number of people diagnosed each year is increasing (CRUK, 2006). The biggest risk factor for cancer is age, and an ageing population means that there will be increasing rates of morbidity over the next few decades. Of the 200 or so types of cancer, breast, lung, bowel and prostate account for over half of all new cases. Over one-quarter of all deaths are caused by cancer in the UK, with 154,547 people recorded as dying from it in 2003 (CRUK, 2006). Cancer mortality rates have dropped by 11 per cent over the last ten years, with significant decreases in the mortality rates for cancers of the cervix, stomach, bowel, lung and breast. The main reasons for falls in mortality are the primary prevention of cancer, earlier detection and better treatment (CRUK, 2006). Overall, breast cancer is the most common cancer in the UK, despite the fact that it is rare in men.

Lung is the most common cancer in men. In 2003 there were 19,806 deaths from lung cancer in men in the UK (CRUK, 2006). Prostate cancer is the second most common cause of cancer death in males, accounting for 13 per cent of male deaths from cancer in 2003. Over 92 per cent of deaths from prostate cancer occur in men aged 65 and over (CRUK, 2006). For women in the UK there are similar numbers of deaths from lung and breast cancer. In 2003, lung cancer was the most common cause of death, responsible for 13,630 deaths in women, compared with 12,614 deaths from breast cancer. Deaths from breast, lung and large bowel cancer together account for nearly half of all female deaths from cancer (CRUK, 2006).

Whilst rates of morbidity are broadly similar in the UK to those in other richer European countries, patterns indicate that survival rates are lower in the UK (Department of Health, 2000). This, it would seem, is partly because patients tend to be at a more advanced stage of the disease by the time they are treated. The DoH suggests that this is probably because patients are not certain when to go to their GP about possible symptoms; GPs have difficulty identifying those at highest risk; and because of the time taken in NHS hospitals to progress from the first appointment through to diagnostic tests to treatment (Department of Health, 2000).

Variation in the quality and provision of NHS cancer services across the country means that not all patients are getting the optimal treatment for their particular condition. Decades of underinvestment have severely restricted NHS cancer services, and it has come under increased pressure to adopt new ways of working and fully exploit new treatment methods to keep NHS cancer services at the forefront of international progress (see Department of Health, 2000). Equipment is out of date and is often incapable of delivering state-of-the-art procedures for diagnosis and treatment, and the NHS has too few cancer specialists of every type. For example, the United Kingdom has around eight oncologists per one million population, less than half that in other comparable European countries (Department of Health, 2000). And there has been a failure to modernise services by adopting new ways of treating patients.

The provision of cancer care is by no means linear across the population despite a largely public-health system in the UK. Social inequality in the context of healthcare provision has been well documented. Socioeconomic status, gender, age, ethnicity and geographic location have been just some of the factors that have been shown to mediate access to, and experience of, primary and tertiary care (e.g. Cancer Research Campaign, 1999; Macleod *et al.*, 2000). Clear differentiation exists, for example, in men's access to primary care and, indeed, the discrepancies in the health outcomes between working-class and middle-class children. There is no doubt that demographic factors mediate everything from morbidity and mortality to treatment by healthcare professionals within healthcare settings.

CAM and cancer

Despite the difficulties in defining CAM outlined above, we can provide some indication of the extent of usage. Bringing together 26 surveys from 13 countries, Ernst and Cassileth (1998) found that on average 31.4 per cent of cancer patients use CAM therapies, ranging from 7 to 64 per cent. UK surveys show similar figures, with over 30 per cent of people with cancer reporting use of CAM (Lewith *et al.*, 2002; Rees *et al.*, 2000). Results between types of cancer are also variable. In a recent study, Scott *et al.* (2005) surveyed 127 adult patients with a diagnosis of cancer from both Scotland and England. CAM use was reported by 29 per cent of the sample. The use of relaxation, meditation and the use of medicinal teas were the most frequently used therapies. A study by Harris *et al.* (2003) of 1,077 Welsh cancer patients found that 49.6 per cent of participants had used at least one type of CAM during the past 12 months and 16.4 per cent had consulted a CAM practitioner.

Morris *et al.* (2000) found that breast cancer patients were far more likely to be consistent users compared with those with other tumour sites, suggestive of variability between patients with different types of cancer (see Fulder, 1996) and/or according to gender. Although little research has been done to tease out such issues, it seems possible that type of cancer, demographics, available treatments, symptoms, rate of progression and the experimental trial programmes available to patients may each have an influence on patients' preferences for CAM and/or biomedical treatment.

CAM, cancer and health policy

Given the high levels of patient support and demand for CAMs, one would expect a general momentum toward merging CAM and biomedicine in policy, if not in practice. However, policy in the area of integrative cancer care has been limited, despite recent political pressure (House of Lords, 2000). The Department of Health has implicitly (and indirectly) attempted to promote a more diverse, integrative and patient-centred approach to cancer care (e.g. Department of Health, 2000, 2004; Tavares, 2003), whilst largely avoiding direct calls for the integration of CAM into the NHS. Those calls for integration that have occurred are still *rigidly* centred on the creation of a biomedical-type evidence base as key for progress to occur (e.g. House of Lords, 2000). In fact, integration, whilst still on the DoH agenda, has largely been a rhetorical device rather than an active plan for grassroots change. The reasons for this are deeply embedded in the issues examined in the following chapters. The powerful lobbying of such organisations as the British

Medical Association (BMA), the Royal College of Physicians (RCP) and other biomedically situated stakeholders has prevented advocates within the political arena from pushing through substantial policy change. However, the political climate is such that pressure is mounting for greater progress to be made, a driving force behind the funding for the study examined in this book. What is certain is that lack of public provision is feeding into a divide in CAM utilisation according to a range of demographic factors, including those discussed below.

Social inequality in cancer care: a focus on factors mediating CAM use

Existing research suggests that, as in other facets of healthcare delivery, gender, socioeconomic status and geographical location may each have an impact on use of and experiences of CAMs (Fouladbakhsh *et al.*, 2005).

As an increasingly significant aspect of patient care, and particularly palliative care (Beider, 2005; Tavares, 2003), equity in access to CAM warrants significant exploration. Moreover, the ways in which patient characteristics influence experiences of disease and treatment processes needs exploration in the context of CAM. Key issues that have hitherto received little attention are: (1) how do gender, socioeconomic status and geographic location impact (if indeed at all) on access to and experiences of CAM; (2) what belief systems and social processes underlie differentiation; and (3) how might patterns of differentiation adversely affect (or indeed benefit) certain patient groups?

Gender and CAM

Gender inequality in UK cancer services is well documented and there exists a considerable body of literature on gender mediating health outcomes more broadly. For example, men have a significantly lower level of awareness of the specific risks to their health compared with women (Court, 1995) and they are generally more resistant than women to seeking help for serious medical problems (Bradlow *et al.*, 1992; Cameron and Bernardes, 1998; Tudiver and Talbot, 1999). Men are generally less able to recognise physical and emotional distress, are less likely to seek help (Harrison *et al.*, 1995; Krizek *et al.*, 1999; R. White, 2002) and are more likely than women to dismiss physical changes and/or problematic symptoms. Men are overrepresented relative to women with regard to certain health problems; for example, they have higher rates of ischemic heart disease, suicide, lung cancer and more car accidents. But how does this feed into CAM-related behaviour (if at all).

Perhaps unsurprisingly, studies of CAM usage have also indicated potential differences in use by women versus men (Fouladbakhsh *et al.*, 2005). For example, compared with males, females were five times more likely to see an 'alternative provider' and about twice as likely to use 'mental' therapies or supplements (see Patterson *et al.*, 2002; and also Adams *et al.*, 2005; Girgis *et al.*, 2005). Certainly, in wider culture CAM has been viewed as intersecting with notions of femininity; indeed, there has been far greater advocacy of CAM in women's magazines and in women's health networks than in other areas of society. Arguments have also been made for the congruence of the CAM 'life world' and elements of feminism (A. Scott, 1998). However, hitherto no study has examined gender differentiation in attitudes towards CAM amongst male and female cancer patients (and particularly in the context of a variety of disease types).

Socioeconomic status, access to cancer care and CAM consumption

There is a significant body of research illustrating ongoing inequality in access to biomedical cancer services and poorer health outcomes for marginalised patient groups. Recent research has shown that people who are from deprived backgrounds are more likely to develop many types of cancers and once diagnosed will have lower chances of survival (Quinn *et al.*, 2001). For example, women with breast cancer who are from deprived areas have significantly lower survival rates than those from affluent areas (Cancer Research Campaign, 1999; Macleod *et al.*, 2000). Prostate cancer shows similar patterns, with studies revealing significant gradients in survival with socioeconomic deprivation. For example, in 1986–90 the one-year survival for prostate cancer was higher by 4 percentage points in men living in the more affluent areas than in those in the most deprived; the five-year survival was 3 points higher (Quinn and Babb, 2002). Patients with bowel cancer who have lower incomes also tend to have a poorer quality of life (Ramsey *et al.*, 2002). Research also shows that patients who are of lower socioeconomic status will ask fewer questions and gain less access to patient support services (i.e. those that often provide free CAM services).

CAM consumption is still largely privately funded and thus access is also linked with socioeconomic status. In their study of selected CAMs, Thomas *et al.* (2001) found that total out-of-pocket expenditure on six established therapies (i.e. acupuncture, chiropractic, homoeopathy, hypnotherapy, medical herbalism and osteopathy) was around £450 million in the UK, and £580 million when reflexology and aromatherapy were included. As a result, income differentials mean certain groups within the UK population have access to CAM services whereas others do not.

Studies also suggest that spending is higher amongst cancer patients than other patient groups. A recent survey (n = 1077) found a median spending of £28 a month on practitioner therapies, £16 on techniques and £10 on diets and supplements (Molassiotis *et al.*, 2006). It seems that cancer increases spending, with a study showing that gynaecologic oncology patients use CAM significantly more than gynaecology patients (66 per cent vs 52 per cent), with a mean total expenditure of US$711 per annum versus US$622 by gynaecology patients (Von Gruenigen *et al.*, 2001). The simple fact that the majority of CAMs are purchased privately necessarily produces a barrier for lower-income populations. We wanted to explore whether such processes influence access to and perceptions of CAM in the UK.

Geographic location and equity

There exist important spatial inequalities in the UK in terms of who gets cancer and what happens to them when they do. The Department of Health acknowledges that cancer patients in different parts of the country receive varying quality and types of treatment (Department of Health, 2000). As such, there is some concern regarding the health and wellbeing of patients living in rural or less central locations (Baird *et al.*, 2000). This potential stratification is not *necessarily* tied to geographical stratification in socio-economic status but rather inconsistencies in the distribution in cancer facilities across the UK (and, of course, processes of centralisation). This relates to CAM in that the majority of CAM services provided *free of charge* by the NHS (or on behalf of the NHS by the volunteer sector) are located in major urban locations, and often in the major teaching hospitals. This can create significant inequality in terms of patient access to CAM therapies.

It should be noted that recent research internationally has indicated that interest in and usage of CAM in rural areas may be higher, in some cases, than in urban locations (Adams *et al.*, 2003; Wilkinson and Simpson, 2001). However, there has been little research done on the impact of geography or hospital site on access to services.

Other potential sites of differentiation

Although these are not focused on in this book, predictors of CAM therapy use also include younger age and higher education (Alferi *et al.*, 2001; Burstein *et al.*, 1999; M. Lee *et al.*, 2000; Richardson *et al.*, 2000). Variation in CAM use by ethnicity has been documented in cancer and general populations (Alferi *et al.*, 2001; Barnes *et al.*, 2004; M. Lee *et al.* 2000). Disease type also presents as a potential site for differentiation. For example, in a study of Canadian women with breast cancer Boon *et al.* (2000) found that 67 per cent of breast cancer patients use CAM therapies – significantly more than the figure reported for many other patient groups. Morris *et al.* (2000) investigated the hypothesis that use of CAM therapies differed between patients with breast cancer and those with other primary tumour sites (n = 617) and found that breast cancer patients were far more likely to be consistent users compared with those having other tumour sites, suggestive of variability between patients with different types of cancer.

Despite the rather concerning patterns outlined above, and despite social differentiation in access to CAM, there is very little sociologically informed research on *why* use of and perceptions of CAM may be mediated by patient demographics. Moreover, how patients get access to CAM knowledge and pathways in CAM services is also largely unknown.

Pathways to CAM: self-help and the information age

A key issue in addressing the support needs of patients with cancer is the quality of information they receive and also the types of sources used to gain access to cancer- and treatment-related information (e.g. Broom, 2006a; Carlsson, 2000). As CAM becomes an increasingly important facet of many cancer patients' experiences of disease and treatment processes, the actual sources of CAM knowledge become increasingly critical in shaping patient decision-making. Who provides cancer patients with CAM information in particular? Previous research by the authors has illustrated the vital role played by patient support groups in guiding patients to CAM (see Chatwin and Tovey, 2004; Tovey, 2003; Tovey *et al.*, 2007). But what other sources of information are used to access CAM knowledge, as only a minority of cancer patients utilise face-to-face support groups?

Existing studies show that cancer patients use many different sources of information to access details of their disease and available therapeutic options. For example, Carlsson (2000) found that cancer patients use a range of sources, including the Internet, telephone helplines, medical books, other patients, friends, television and radio, and newspapers. Studies have also shown the Internet to be popular amongst patients (e.g. Broom, 2005). Although results have been mixed in terms of patient preferences for, say, books versus the Internet, Basch *et al.* (2004) found that print resources, such as books and pamphlets, were used *more often* than the Internet. Telephone resources were used substantially less often than either the Internet or print resources. Basch *et al.* (2004) also found that print-resource users most commonly sought information on cancer diagnosis and treatment, but these patients were *more* likely to research nutrition than Internet users. However, both Internet and traditional print media users investigated CAM (Basch *et al.*, 2004). This suggests that information source selection may be highly differentiated according to the type of information needed and the stage in the treatment process (see also Broom, 2005).

The Internet certainly represents the most fundamental change in information exchange and retrieval of the twentieth and twenty-first centuries and potentially opens up the possibility of a 'virtual' liberalisation of health information (Broom, 2005; Broom, 2006a). Prior to the emergence of the Internet, medical knowledge was largely confined to the realm of the medical professional, allowing relatively little public access to and scrutiny of expert knowledges and practices. Furthermore, access to CAM knowledge was limited to self-help books and the support and advice of individual practitioners, restricting the degree to which patients could become informed about different paradigms of care and the various treatment options available to them. As such, the Internet could potentially play a key role as a porthole to non-biomedical therapeutic options (S. Fox, 2005) and, furthermore, it could have a democratising impact in a socio-cultural context hitherto dominated by a biomedical view of illness (Anderson *et al.*, 2003; N. Fox *et al.*, 2005;

Hardey, 1999). However, despite considerable conjecture, there has been virtually no work done on the Internet as a pathway to CAM for cancer patients and none that is sociologically informed. Thus, in Chapter 3 we critically examine the Internet as a source of information and support for cancer patients, looking at both benefits and limitations of the online medium.

Cancer clinicians' attitudes towards CAM

The issue of how CAM is dealt with within the medical consultation is of critical importance to patient experience of disease and treatment processes. However, there is emerging and concerning evidence that use of CAM is not discussed openly between patients and their physicians and that CAM-related issues can create problematic dynamics within medical consultations. Tasaki *et al.* (2002) suggest that indifference toward CAM, concerns over evidence (on the part of the doctor) and patients' expectation of negativity each contribute to difficulties within medical consultations. However, as we explore in detail in Chapter 3, there is significant differentiation in how doctors view CAM (Astin *et al.*, 1998), with some supporting certain CAMs and thus being willing to refer patients on to CAM therapists. In their study, for example, J. Bernstein and Shuval (1997) found that nearly all of the physicians they interviewed would (or do) refer patients to CAM practitioners (see also Goldszmidt *et al.*, 1995; A. White *et al.*, 1997).

Studies based on the self-reported beliefs and approaches of doctors are necessarily limited in that such accounts do not *necessarily* reflect what happens in practice. Indeed, perceptions of professional practice and approach should be viewed with some scepticism (see Hirschkorn and Bourgeault, 2005). Hence, in Chapter 3 we explore cancer patients' *own* accounts of their doctors' and nurses' views of and advice about CAM in the context of cancer care. Although this still only provides a retrospective account of interpersonal dynamics (rather than actual recordings of consultations), it does provide valuable insight into how cancer patients are experiencing their interactions with their consultant oncologists.

Whilst oncology as a medical specialty has remained highly sceptical toward CAM, cancer nursing has positioned itself quite differently, with important implications for patient care and inter-professional dynamics. Previous literature in the area has pointed to the rather different relationship of certain facets of nursing to CAM, with nurses frequently being presented as patient-centred rather than disease-centred and holistic rather than mechanistic in approach. As such, nursing has taken a rather different trajectory to medicine in terms of how to manage the increased presence (and popularity of) CAM (see Boschma, 1994). The increasing presence of CAM is thus potentially *less* challenging to the nursing profession than it is to certain elements of the medical profession. Whilst more research needs to be done – and Chapter 3 contributes significantly to knowledge in this area – it seems likely that nursing as a profession will play a key role in mediating the interface of CAM and biomedicine. Given levels of advocacy amongst the nursing community, nurses are well placed to play such a role (e.g. Chong, 2006; Lengacher *et al.*, 2006). Although there has been very little research in this area, it seems possible that CAM advocacy and, indeed, some degree of alignment of nursing as a profession with CAM may have the advantage, for nurses, of further differentiating them from medicine and thus feeding into ongoing processes of distinction between nursing and medicine (Tovey and Adams, 2003). In Chapter 3 we critically engage with these inter- and intra-professional issues, further highlighting the (emerging) complex relationships between nursing, CAM and biomedicine.

The sociology of CAM

Theorising CAM and the individual

The question of *why* patients are increasingly utilising CAM therapies has been under-researched; hence the development of the project examined here and the writing of this book. However, there has been considerable theorising by sociologists as to the underlying causes driving increased CAM consumption. Of particular interest to sociologists has been whether public interest in (and usage of CAM) represents a wider cultural shift, and what such patterns say about the nature of the individual, the subject and contemporary therapeutic culture. There has been increased questioning of why, after decades of deference to biomedical expertise, significant numbers of people *seem* to be wavering in their support for biomedicine, and biomedical cancer care in particular. This is despite some significant successes in biomedical cancer treatment and prevention. For example, nine out of ten children recover from Hodgkin's disease, whereas 30 years ago only about half survived (NCI, 1999). Moreover, up to 70 per cent of *all* children with cancer can now be cured, with childhood leukaemia (once a certain death sentence) having an 80 per cent cure rate (NCCF, 2003).

Despite these advances in biomedicine, patients (and cancer patients in particular) seem increasingly inclined to use non-biomedical therapeutics either in combination with or as an alternative to biomedical care. To make sense of these intriguing societal patterns, sociologists have attempted to connect CAM consumption (theoretically) to wider socio-cultural shifts. What follows is a fairly brief outline of the most popular strains of social theory as applied to CAM.

The postmodernisation thesis has been popular over the last decade amongst some sociologists as an explanation for the increased presence of CAM. CAM use, it is argued, is indicative of a broader postmodernisation of social life (e.g. Bakx, 1991; Eastwood, 2000; Rayner and Easthope, 2001; Siahpush, 1998), which is contributing to: the fragmentation of experience, consumerism, individualisation and the aestheticisation of social life. In the context of healthcare, dominant discourses (such as the biomedical model outlined above) are subsumed by subjective individualised knowledges that inform social practices and identity work. The pre-eminence of biomedical conceptions of disease is thus rejected in place of an individualised, subjectified approach to illness whereby narrative and individual perception reign supreme. While this theoretical position in relation to CAM has been quite popular and widely drawn on, it has lacked empirical testing and, as seen in Chapter 1, is at best of limited relevance to cancer patients' lived experiences.

Theorisations of late modernity, as in other areas of sociology, have been viewed as potentially useful in explaining the increased presence of non-biomedical therapeutics (Low, 2004; Tovey *et al.*, 2001). Such work has drawn on authors like Beck (1992) and Giddens (1990, 1991), who have focused on increased reflexivity in modern societies and the tendency of 'consumers' to be more critical of expert knowledges. This body of work espoused the notion of reflexive modernisation, which, among other things, refers to the questioning of the process of modernisation in terms of the array of risks one is presented with (Beck, 1992). The result, some argue, is a fixation with risk within public debate, and concern about risks in people's private lives (for discussion of this, see Lupton, 1995, 1997, 1999). Such arguments also relate to changes in the public perception of medical knowledge and expertise. The result of processes of reflexive modernisation, it is argued, is that people have become more sceptical about the judgements or advice of (scientific) experts (Lupton and Tulloch, 2002), actively assessing the merits of particular claims. This, in turn, it has been postulated, has opened up the potential for the proliferation of CAM – a backlash against the perceived failings of science and biomedical technologies (Kaptchuk and Eisenberg, 1998).

Others have pursued less grandiose conceptualisations of CAM consumption and experience, suggesting that non-biomedical therapeutics offer a more holistic, subjectified form of patient care that provides a valuable addition to biomedical, physiologically focused cancer treatments (e.g. Bishop and Yardley, 2004). Related work has examined the degree to which CAM use represents a significant shift in conceptions of disease and selfhood. In particular, the notion of *wellbeing* has emerged recently as a potentially useful concept for characterising what CAM offers to the individual. Departing from biomedical notions of being 'cured', 'healthy' or 'disease free', wellbeing encapsulates notions of authenticity, recognition and self-determination, restructuring 'health' as a subjective and individualised process (Bishop and Yardley, 2004; Sointu, 2006; see also Wray, 2007). CAM use is thus conceptualised as a project of the self – an individual search for recognition as an authentic self that is both 'discovered' by the individual and shaped by the nature of individual therapeutic practices.

Social theorisations of wellbeing have emphasised the limitations of biomedical conceptions of disease and health, and are thus, in part, a natural conceptual extension of the depersonalisation (e.g. McClean, 2005) and deindividualisation (e.g. Anspach, 1988) theses. These two latter arguments refer broadly to processes by which many biomedical clinicians abstract from the individual through speech (i.e. referring to 'the patient'), technologies (i.e. the person as a biomedicalised image), statistical probabilities (i.e. the group rather than individual), units of analysis (e.g. genes/cellular) and so on, rather than acknowledging the individual subject. This is seen to alienate the patient from treatment processes – perhaps even resulting in the need for alternative therapeutic options.

As illustrated above, sociological theory as applied to individual engagement with CAM has tended to reify broader socio-cultural shifts in relation to individual choice, conceptions of disease and lay/expert relations. Rather than reflecting broad paradigmatic change, we argue in the following chapters (see particularly Chapter 1) that the increasing presence of CAM in cancer care is complex and differentiated.

Theorising CAM and the medical profession

The majority of social theorising around CAM has been regarding the inter- and intra-professional boundary disputes between CAM and biomedicine (e.g. Broom, 2002; Broom and Tovey, 2007; Dew, 1997, 1998, 2000, 2000a; Hirschkorn and Bourgeault, 2005; Kelner *et al.*, 2004; Mizrachi *et al.*, 2005; Saks, 1992, 1994, 1996, 1998; Tovey and Adams, 2001). Much early work in the sociology of CAM focused on notions of medical dominance (see Willis, 2006) and the hegemonic potential of biomedicine's virtual monopoly over healthcare delivery. Studies of CAM (particularly chiropractic) and midwifery were used to illustrate the strong political power of biomedicine in shaping the nature and delivery of primary healthcare (e.g. Dew, 2000, 2000a). Part of this work aimed to illustrate that healthcare delivery was not, and is not, purely based on what is 'effective' or 'efficacious'. Rather, what constitutes these very notions is a mix of the physiological, contextual, ideological and political. Paradigmatic basis, it has been argued, has been fundamental in assessing the legitimacy of a therapeutic intervention, and such arguments regularly underlie sociological critiques of medical power and dominance (Willis, 1989). This biomedical trajectory of relative clinical autonomy has necessarily involved the deployment of a variety of discursive and regulatory means of maintaining control of primary healthcare delivery, particularly in relation to CAM and midwifery. We have witnessed the constraints imposed on the encroachment of non-biomedical therapeutics into primary care. Empirical studies have illustrated the complex subordination of various actors increasingly operating in hospital systems (e.g. midwives) as well as those operating within the community (i.e. CAM practitioners) (e.g. Kelner *et al.*, 2004).

In recent years, although the biomedical community has to a certain degree maintained much of this control, a relative waning in the dominance and professional autonomy of biomedicine has driven some sociologists to reflect on whether previous conceptualisations of medical dominance are actually relevant to contemporary healthcare organisation (Broom, 2006). Such debates have been prompted by such things as increased public scepticism towards scientific and technological development, lack of recent progress in biomedicine in the treatment and prevention of disease and increased use of non-biomedical therapeutics (e.g. Calnan *et al.*, 2005). Moreover, structural processes occurring within medicine, such as increased manageralism, have prompted questions regarding the relevance of previous conceptualisations of the relationship of the biomedical community to other professional groups, their patients, the state or indeed the public (Gray, 2002). This has, in part, resulted in the development of theorisations of a so-called waning in medical power and autonomy, including the deprofessionalisation and proletarianisation theses. Proletarianisation represents the process whereby organisational and managerial changes divest professionals of the control they have enjoyed over their work (Hardey, 1999). Deprofessionalisation, in the context of the medical profession, is associated with a demystification of medical expertise and increasing lay scepticism about health professionals. This process of deprofessionalisation is seen to result from reductions in monopolisation of esoteric knowledge, autonomy in work performance and authority over clients (Gray, 2002; Haug, 1973, 1988; Lewis *et al.*, 2003).

Given such arguments about medical power and authority, does the persistence of CAM present a potential challenge to, and threaten the reconfiguration of, established biomedical organisational culture? Does the potential (and actual) introduction of CAMs for cancer patients offer a challenge to the symbolic power of the medical profession (Boon *et al.*, 2004), potentially reconstructing them as one of a number of cancer clinicians and, furthermore, potentially questioning the central tenets of their epistemological/ ideological position? Would the increased integration of CAM within the NHS contribute, among other factors, to this so-called deprofessionalisation of biomedicine? Certainly, the proliferation of CAM has to a certain degree catalysed a movement towards a market or consumerist model of healthcare, increasing the range of options available to consumers, encouraging patients to question biomedical advice, and potentially challenging the monopoly of biomedicine in healthcare delivery (Bombardieri and Easthope, 2000). Furthermore, the increased consumption of CAM by patients has been seen as part of a broader movement towards a questioning of the benefits of the primacy of biomedicine in health provision and as a challenge to doctors' clinical authority (e.g. Lupton, 1997).

However, we argue in the following chapters that a more nuanced approach is needed to examine how CAM is viewed, utilised and managed by different actors; what position CAMs are allowed to occupy within particular organisational settings; and the mechanics of how such roles are negotiated, or indeed enforced. Pursuing a dualistic conception of inter-professional dynamics as about dominance/subordination, power/oppression, tends to engender a monolithic, binary view of professional positionings. This despite the fact that, as explored in the following chapters, recent changes that have been occurring in medicine are complex, highly differentiated and indeed context specific. What is needed, in our view, is a critical sociology of the roles and positions of biomedicine that accurately represents the differentiated and evolving nature of inter-professional and lay/expert dynamics.

In particular, insight is needed into patients' and clinicians' relationships with, and responses to, CAM to actually discover what is occurring at the point of service delivery. We know little about whether (and in what ways) CAMs and biomedicine are being shaped by processes of integration, and the implications for professional identities and therapeutic processes. In order to engage with such issues, in this book we move past oversimplified binary constructions of the relationship between CAM and biomedicine to examine the mechanisms through which integration is managed, reflecting on the implications for CAM in cancer care, within and between different organisa-tional contexts. We move beyond binary analyses of CAM and biomed-icine emphasising the complexity of grassroots organisational processes and the importance of intra-professional differentiation (e.g. Timmermans and Kolker, 2004). In effect, this moves the argument forward from binary con-ceptions of inter- (and intra-)professional and expert/lay dynamics to a more complex view whereby actors evolve in relation to each other, enlisting par-ticular things in their attempts to reinforce or bolster their position within a given network. Much attention has been paid to methods of exclusion or appropriation, and little to the ways in which the interconnections between entities are involved in the production of these very things.

On methods and methodology

The methodology for the project examined in this book draws on the interpretive traditions within qualitative research, incorporating aspects of grounded theory, symbolic interactionalism and phenomenological approaches to social research. This broadly defined interpretivist or con-structivist tradition is associated with such authors as Glaser and Strauss (1967), Berger and Luckman (1967), Geertz (1973), Lofland and Lofland (1984) and Rubin and Rubin (1995), to name just a few. Rather than seeking to measure or categorise behaviour or attitudes (typical of more positivistic survey/questionnaire-based approaches), we sought to establish an in-depth understanding of the experiences of the respondents and the meanings within their stories (Wainwright, 1997). It was about how the patients, doctors and nurses construct their worlds (Charmaz, 1990) and, in particular, how they made sense of the role (and impacts) of CAM within these worlds. As such, we focus in the following chapters on their interpretations and the meanings in their stories, pursuing an analysis which maintains a constructivist onto-logical position that actors actively *negotiate meaning* (see Broom, 2005c). As such, we view the accounts presented as snapshots of the process of constructing and contesting social 'facts' (e.g. what constitutes 'CAM', 'effectiveness', 'evidence' or 'legitimacy').

The advantage of flexible, descriptive, qualitative analysis such as that employed here is that one can produce observations that demand the creation of new ideas and categories that might not emerge in more structured analyses (Charmaz, 1990; Ezzy, 2002; Strauss and Corbin, 1990). As such, it is possible to adjust one's approach in response to data which may contradict one's initial assumptions or theories on, for example, why patients utilise CAM or how integration of CAM may be viewed by differently positioned cancer clinicians (see Broom, 2005c). By giving attention to those cases that do not fit, to those strategic actions that do not at first make sense, to those incongruities so often bypassed by quantitative methods, we see the complexity of social processes (Gubrium and Holstein, 1997). In addition, the area of CAM and cancer is hugely under-researched and, as a consequence, relatively little was known about the study's research questions. An exploratory, interpretivist and flexible approach is particularly appropriate in these circumstances (Bryman and Burgess, 1994). Thus, we decided on a multiphased qualitative design, employing in-depth interviews and solicited diary/unstructured interview case studies. This combination allowed us to select participants according to specific criteria (such as stage of cancer) as well as providing the means to trace processes of decision-making within the context of individuals' lives. We completed in-depth interviews with 80 cancer patients and 31 cancer clinicians, as well as eight one-month diary case studies. What follows is a description of these two distinct but interconnected study arms.

Phase 1: in-depth qualitative interviews with patients and clinicians

Patient interviews

After ethics approval was secured, we approached three NHS teaching hospitals and one partially NHS-funded hospice involved in cancer and palliative care services in the North of England. Two cancer/palliative care specialists and a CAM coordinator at the hospice who had formed part of the project team assisted with recruitment. Patients were recruited via posters placed in oncology wards and patient information and support centres. The final sample included 80 cancer patients with a good distribution of ages from 20 to 87 and representation from all major cancer types. We deliberately sampled to include high numbers of CAM users to gain insight into decision-making, experiences of disease and treatment processes, and the importance of such things as 'evidence' and 'risk/harm' therein. We also included around 15 per cent non-CAM users to gain some insight into perceptions from a range of usage levels (from exclusively CAM to no CAM usage to this point in time). Thus, this is a study of predominantly CAM users who are cancer patients rather than a representative sample of all cancer patients; this recognition informs our analysis in the following chapters. One-third of the participants were male and two-thirds were female. Given the high proportion of female CAM users we expected to get more female participants. The number of excerpts presented in the results broadly reflects this differential. Of the sample, 68 were white British. The remaining were Irish (4), Indian (2), Italian (2), German (2) and Eastern European (2). We included the following patient groups in the sample: patients receiving potentially curative treatment; patients who had received potentially curative treatment and were clinically free of disease; patients with metastatic disease who were receiving or had been recommended biomedical cancer treatment; and patients with advanced disease who were receiving or were candidates for palliative care. The patients were fairly evenly distributed between these categories, although patients with metastatic disease formed the largest group.

All the respondents were interviewed for between one and two hours either in their own homes, in their oncology ward, at the hospice or at the authors' university. With the permission of the participant, the interviews were tape recorded and subsequently fully transcribed. The interviews were relatively unstructured, exploring such things as perceptions and experiences of CAM and biomedical cancer care; the role and nature of 'evidence' in disease experience and treatment decision-making; pathways to CAM and key sources of CAM information and support; cancer clinicians' attitudes to CAM and the doctor/patient relationship; and individual beliefs about CAM integration in cancer care. The aim was to achieve a detailed understanding of the varying positions adhered to, and to locate these within an appreciation of broader underlying beliefs and/or agendas. The approach we used was developmental, in that knowledge generated in the early interviews was challenged by, compared with and built upon by later ones.

There were numerous ethical considerations within the research process that are quite particular to research involving cancer patients, including limiting potential physical discomfort or emotional distress (see Broom, 2006b). There were times during the interviews that participants were emotional and we ensured that they were able to stop the interview and withdraw from the study, and where necessary we gave details of patient-support organisations they could get in contact with. In actuality, none of the patients opted to withdraw once the interview had begun. Both the authors were constantly aware of the need to balance the desire of participants to 'give something back' and the need to minimise distress as a result of participation. The interviews with the hospice patients raised quite specific ethical issues. Generally patients in hospice care are within months, if not weeks, of death. After considerable discussion with hospice staff, patients considered cognitively impaired and/or very close to death were not considered for participation. The interviews in the hospice were sometimes cut short so as not to tire the interviewee, and in general the hospice was a challenging place to do interviews for researcher and participant. On several occasions other people in the hospice passed away during an interview; the hospice bell would ring and the person's body would be wheeled through the corridors to be taken away. Although challenging experiences, they were also crucial as they allowed insight into the context in which the stories being told are embedded; thus they contributed significantly to the interpretations offered in the following chapters.

Clinician interviews

We selected two organisations (from those we were recruiting patients from) that would provide us with interesting cases of CAM integration in the UK. These organisations were selected because both have innovative character- istics such as staff involved in high-profile roles in establishing national CAM guidelines and, second, in the case of the hospital, a large support centre located within the hospital providing CAM treatments to cancer patients. The organisations are as follows (see Chapter 3 for more details):

Hospital: The NHS teaching hospital that we examined has one of the largest cancer-treatment facilities in the north of England. It has facilities for providing support and CAM services to cancer patients, through a centre set up and funded by the volunteer sector and located in the centre of the hospital site. This centre offers cancer patients a range of CAMs. The CAM therapists are volunteers, offering, generally, one day a week of their time to provide their therapy free to cancer patients.

Hospice: The hospice we selected provides patients with an array of CAM therapies, including acupuncture, reiki, massage, hypnotherapy, reflex- ology and aromatherapy. The majority of the patients at the hospice are cancer patients. Two palliative care consultants supervise all treatments offered in the hospice. Although the hospice receives some NHS funding, a significant proportion comes from public donations. Thus, there is a degree of autonomy in the hospice movement, resulting, as we see in Chapter 3, in quite different strategies to integrate CAM.

Within these organisations we interviewed 31 key individuals, including 12 medical specialists (i.e. medical oncologists, radiation oncologists, pallia- tive care specialists); 6 specialist cancer and palliative care nurses; 6 CAM therapists (including 2 coordinators); 2 radiologists; 4 specialist cancer and palliative care pharmacists; and 1 specialist palliative care occupational ther- apist. At the time of the interviews the two radiologists were employed by another hospital in the North of England. The interviews were generally between one and two hours long and were recorded and transcribed. The interviews explored how differently positioned cancer clinicians were reacting to, and adapting to, the increasing presence of CAM in NHS cancer ser- vices; the role of CAM in cancer care in their specific organisation context; views about the role of evidence; and beliefs about therapeutic processes in biomedical care and CAM. Examples of the questions asked include: what constitutes evidence in your perspective? How do you personally judge the effectiveness of a treatment? How do you view CAM therapies in relation to evidence? Within your organisation, how is funding secured for

CAM or biomedical treatments and what is the role of evidence within this process?

Phase 2: the solicited diary/unstructured interview

From the 80 NHS cancer patients, we purposively selected eight participants to complete a one-month solicited diary and a follow-up unstructured interview. The basis of the selection was that each could offer insight into issues identified in Phase 1 but which had only partially been explored because of the restricted nature of individual, one-off interviews. Our initial selection of a total of eight participants was reviewed once the diary phase had begun with a view to increasing the number if required. In the event, because of the depth and coverage of the data produced this was deemed unnecessary by the project team at the point of review.

The selection of one month was also kept under review. Longer periods were considered but the need to protect patients from undue stress coupled with the (confirmed) likelihood of producing considerable data meant we opted for a shorted timeframe. Like others who have used diary methods (see Jacelon and Imperio, 2005; Zimmerman and Wieder, 1977), we used face-to-face unstructured interviews for participant checks and elaboration of the diaries. Previous use of this approach suggested that the combination of a solicited diary followed by an unstructured interview focused on the events chronicled in the diary would be an effective method of obtaining rich data (Corti, 1993; see also Broom and Adams, 2007). This diary and interview combination was designed to explore use of, and preferences for, CAM over time and space. The eight participants were selected from the overall sample as they had a range of disease stages and disease types, including those with ovarian cancer (3), breast cancer (2), multiple myloma (1), Hodgkin's (1) and lung cancer (1). We included 2 men and 6 women (broadly proportionate to the gender mix of the overall sample of 80 patients) and a range of ages (25–85). Each participant was a very active CAM user when given the diary; we targeted the more proactive CAM users in order to get a rich data set on experiences of CAM over time.

The one-month diaries were all completed. Seven of the eight patients were interviewed for a second time after completion of the diary. One patient could not be interviewed as he died before the second interview could take place, and his wife was interviewed instead to help make sense of the diary. The aim was for the diaries to be as flexible as possible rather than determinative. At the beginning of each diary we gave the following instructions:

- Be honest about how you feel. If you feel negative or unhappy that's ok but try and explain why.
- We are very interested in how you feel about any conversations/ interactions you have with friends, family, doctors or complementary therapists that are related to your health. Please try and document these as well as the physical effects of the therapies you are taking.

- If you feel unwell, and can't fill in the diary, don't worry, there's always tomorrow!

After analysis of the initial 80 interviews, we developed questions that would tease out issues emerging from the initial data but focus in on process and changes over time. The emphasis, therefore, was on gaining a better understanding of the temporal dimension of cancer and CAM use. We sought to explore such questions as: what are the implications of every-day processes, interactions and treatment cycles for patient perceptions of therapeutic options; and how would symptomatology (e.g. pain, nausea, depression, anxiety, etc.) intersect with perceptions and experiences of CAM? Each day of the diary contained the following open-ended questions, with considerable space for the participant to write their thoughts and experiences:

1   What medications, therapies, or health-related activities have you done/ taken today and how have these affected you physically/ emotionally/ spiritually?
2   Please describe any important events that have occurred today (i.e. medical consultation/ healing session/support group meeting/meeting with family or friends).
3   Could you write down any thoughts or experiences you've had today regarding your health or wellbeing (i.e. thoughts emerging from things such as reading books, meeting friends, searching the Internet and talking with family members)?
4   Please add any other comments that you may feel are important for us to understand your experience today.

Data analysis

As outlined above, the methodology for this project draws on the interpretive traditions within qualitative research, focusing on establishing an in-depth understanding of the experiences of the respondents. Data analysis for Phase 1 and Phase 2 was based on four questions adapted from Charmaz's (1990) approach to social analysis: What is the basis of a particular experience, action, belief, relationship or structure? What do these assume implicitly or explicitly about particular subjects and relationships? Of what larger process is this action/belief etc. a part? What are the implications of such actions/beliefs for particular actors/institutional forms? One of the authors undertook primary analysis; interpretations produced were challenged and tested by the other author; initial interpretations were re-tested against the data and the final understanding of the data, presented here, generated.

Outline of the book

Chapter 1 examines patients' perspectives on the nature of evidence and the degree to which different understandings of evidence inform decision-making about CAM and biomedical cancer treatments. Results illustrate the ways in which these cancer patients' critically engage with questions about the nature of knowledge and the potential pitfalls of science. Their accounts can largely be characterised by a dialectical tension between individuation (espoused by many CAM therapies) and depersonalisation (implicit in biomedical care); a tension mediated by the individual cancer patients' prognosis and age. On the basis of the results we argue for a refocusing of social theory to embrace an understanding of grassroots ontological tensions seen in the experiences of individual cancer patients. The problematic nature of maintaining a narrowly defined 'evidence-base' policy on CAM and cancer is also discussed in light of the data.

Chapter 2 focuses on the role the Internet plays in the context of decisions to use CAM. Analysis of the data departs from previous representations of the Internet as a major source of CAM knowledge and, second, as a major pathway to patients' CAM usage. Moreover, the results highlight the potentially damaging impact of the Internet for some cancer patients. Significant anxiety was evident as patients attempted to processes vast amounts of complex biomedical knowledge and, second, from exposure to negative diagnostic and prognostic information. This was particularly evident in the accounts of the patients who were attempting to embrace alternative therapeutic models; in such cases the Internet was often viewed as a dangerous entity (due to its biomedicalisation) to be avoided. This chapter argues that binary constructions of the Internet as a haven for quackery or the provision of 'quality' biomedical information as 'safe' for patients are at best oversimplistic. We suggest that sociological arguments regarding the democratisation of knowledge, the deprofessionalisation of medicine or linear notions of Internet-based empowerment misrepresent the dominance of biomedical knowledge online and the Internet's role in reinforcing biomedicine's paradigmatic dominance in cancer care.

Chapter 3 examines interviews with medical specialists, nursing staff and CAM therapists in the hospice and the hospital. This chapter focuses on how integration is managed, examining professional boundary disputes and interprofessional dynamics. Discussion focuses on the rhetorical and practical strategies that are employed by a variety of differently positioned interviewees to negotiate the complexities of the interface of CAM and biomedicine. Our analysis shows significant differentiation in how differently positioned cancer clinicians view and utilise the biomedical hierarchy of evidence. We argue that the integration of CAM should not be conceptualised as a mere challenge to biomedicine or as resulting in a linear process of deprofessionalisation. Rather, it should be seen as producing a complex array of processes, including strategic adaptation on the part of medical specialists and NHS organisations.

Chapter 4 examines patient experiences of discussions about CAM with biomedical cancer specialists in this increasingly complex social environment. This chapter addresses three issues: patient experience with cancer specialists; the significance of that experience for patient engagement with CAM; and the nature and significance of inter-professional dynamics. Patients reported three main types of approach by oncologists: explicit or implicit negativity; supportive ambivalence; and pragmatic acceptance. Crucially, patients' accounts suggest that the type of approach adopted influences patient action. Specialist cancer nurses emerged as potentially powerful mediators between oncologists and patients. Despite the apparent potential for influence from multiple information sources and 'experts', on the basis of this study we would argue that oncologists remain crucial to patient engagement with CAM. However, this is not to argue that the influence is a determining one. Where patient and medical perspectives diverge, strategic alignment with specialist nurses may help patients make choices which conflict with perceived advice.

Drawing on data from solicited diaries, Chapter 5 examines individual cancer patients' experiences of CAM over time. Patients recorded their experiences in a one-month diary and participated in a single follow-up unstructured qualitative interview to confirm our interpretations of their written accounts. Our findings suggest that experiences of and perceptions of CAM are variable over time and space and, furthermore, that the everyday act of 'doing CAM' is considerably more problematic than is often reported in face-to-face interview or survey studies. We argue that an emphasis on the temporality of cancer patients' CAM engagement is necessary to access a more nuanced understanding of the lived experiences of cancer patients. The findings also throw further doubt on conceptualisations of CAM use as engendering major paradigmatic cultural shift as indicated in much sociological work hitherto. The seemingly mundane elements of CAM users' day-to-day lives indicate a more differentiated and changeable character to individual engagement with non-biomedical therapeutics, suggesting the need for a reassessment of methodological and theoretical bases to previous CAM sociology.

Chapter 6 examines the assumption of a link between use and support for integration. On the basis of this data collected we argue that: (1) a characterisation of unequivocal cancer patient support for integration (even amongst those who use CAM) is an oversimplification and distortion of the situation; (2) it is inappropriate to conflate 'use' with 'advocacy'; (3) patients' engagement with the idea of integration is complex and multi-layered; and (4) this complexity can be explicated by looking at key dimensions of an integrative process – evidence and risk, cost, and provider legitimacy.

We conclude with a chapter which summarises the key points of the book and draws together its various component parts; themes which cut across the chapters are identified. In this concluding section we also take the opportunity to return to a broader discussion of the value of sociological work in the field which is not tied to immediate and narrow policy objectives. In this context we sketch out an agenda of research priorities for the field, which links with and develops themes discussed in the book.

1 The dialectical tension between individuation and depersonalisation in cancer patients' mediation of therapeutic options

Introduction

As outlined in the Introduction, the potential integration of CAM into the UK cancer services has become a key issue for the UK DoH. However, the movement toward a more rounded, and less exclusively biomedical, approach to cancer care has been slow. Although national cancer policy is increasingly advocating, albeit implicitly, 'integrative' and 'patient-centred' practice (Department of Health, 2000, 2004), a virtual stalemate in the debate about 'evidence' and 'efficacy' has prevented any real progress being made. Many biomedical clinicians and health researchers argue for the development of a biomedical-type evidence base before there is even consideration of using CAM therapies for NHS cancer patients (Ernst, 2001). 'Unproven' therapies, it is argued, should not be offered to patients (House of Lords, 2000) due to risks of potential harm and wasting NHS resources. However, an increasingly popular perspective amongst CAM practitioners, patient groups and some social scientists alike is that professional gate-keeping, paradigmatic incommensurability and restrictive understandings of 'evidence' are the real barriers to state funding of CAM for cancer patients (e.g. Borgerson, 2005; Broom and Tovey, 2007). Moreover, cancer patients themselves are increasingly choosing treatments regardless of their clinical 'efficacy' (e.g. Lewith *et al.*, 2002), suggesting the pursuit of evidence-based medicine (EBM) in cancer care may have little resonance with many patients' experiences.

There are considerable gaps in our knowledge regarding the appeal of CAM and the ways in which CAM may problematise biomedical understandings of effectiveness. Research (especially in relation to cancer) has tended merely to describe patterns of usage rather than empirically and theoretically explore the beliefs and understandings underpinning use. Little research has been done on why cancer patients use CAM and their perceptions of 'scientific' evidence in treatment decision-making. Sociological analyses have also tended to focus on clinicians' perspectives (be they CAM and biomedical) on evidence and evidence-based medicine (e.g. Broom and Tovey, 2007a; Pope, 2003).

As such, the aim of this chapter is to provide an examination of cancer patients' perspectives on the 'nature' of evidence and the degree to which different understandings of evidence inform decision-making about CAM and biomedicine. In addressing this aim, the chapter engages with issues of wider relevance, including the empirically grounded critique of social theory and the complexities surrounding the move to evidence-based practice. The current trajectory of DoH policy with regard to cancer care is toward the creation of a biomedical-type evidence base to inform both decisions on funding and patients' decision-making. This, it is argued, would ensure that patients would be able to avoid 'ineffective treatments'. However, as we demonstrate in this chapter, while cancer patients may understand the nature of 'scientific' evidence *per se*, and its usefulness in certain scenarios, many *also* perceive scientific evidence to be inadequate for measuring 'effectiveness' and thus predicting how their body will respond to treatment.

In fact, the accounts presented below suggest that cancer patients may desire elements of the therapeutic process that currently are not adequately acknowledged and promoted by existing biomedical measures of effectiveness; such things include the need for self-determination, and recognition of individual subjectivity and agency in treatment processes. These very needs, we argue here, are heightened for some patients through processes of depersonalisation within biomedical contexts, creating a dialectical tension, for patients, between individuation (e.g. agency, self-responsibility and individualised healing) and depersonalisation (e.g. cure rates and statistical probabilities), within which individual prognosis and age play an important role. On the basis of these findings we argue in this chapter for a refocusing of social theory to embrace an understanding of grassroots ontological tensions seen in the experiences of individual cancer patients. We also warn against employing a narrowly defined 'evidence-base' policy on CAM and cancer.

EBM and patients

Debate about EBM, and more recently, evidence-based practice (EBP), has been a dominant feature of professional discourse over the last decade or so. The randomised controlled trial (RCT) and meta-analysis in systematic review have become, at least in principle, the only 'legitimate' means of producing knowledge of the body, disease and treatment processes. 'Evidence', in state policy, has become inextricably tied to a particular methodological design (and epistemological position); other forms of knowledge production have little explicit influence on UK cancer policy. Moreover, it is becoming increasingly apparent that patient needs may not be easily reconciled with EBM policy, cancer care being a prime example. Increasing pressure is being put on oncology departments to provide psychosocial interventions and CAM therapies for patients undergoing treatment. This process has been hindered by hospital-based oncology services having been traditionally focused on cure rates and disease reduction. As a result, there are still only limited resources available for emotional, social and spiritual aspects of cancer care.

EBM, as a policy framework, is often cited as a justification for the exclusion of CAM practices. However, critics argue that EBM is, ideologically, highly restrictive, a threat to doctor/patient communication and to the value of individual clinical judgement (e.g. Mykhalovskiy, 2003). Moreover, it may be the case that, increasingly, biomedical views on what constitutes effectiveness play less of a role in patients' treatment choices and differ considerably from the views of many CAM practitioners (Borgerson, 2005). Thus, the question of the barriers posed by EBM, and its therapeutic legitimacy, is a central issue that needs examining in terms of the potential role of CAM in cancer care.

CAM and evidence

Critiques of biomedicine have often centred on the highly positivist ontological framework imposed by the biomedical model and the epistemological biases inherent in knowledge produced through RCTs (Borgerson, 2005). The RCT, some argue, provides a highly restrictive view of the therapeutic process and is gauged towards measuring reductionistic notions of effectiveness. Through the imposition of a disease-centred (rather than patient-centred) framework (as outlined in the Introduction), CAMs have been viewed by many as 'unproven', whereas, it is often argued by advocates, the therapeutic processes involved in CAM practices cannot be adequately captured in a positivist framework (e.g. Borgerson, 2005). This has led some to focus on more patient-centred and subjective gauges of validity, including notions of 'wellbeing', 'healing' and achieving 'balance'.

Efforts to prompt biomedical organisations and clinicians to engage critically in debates about 'evidence' production and address complex ideological and paradigmatic issues have been largely unsuccessful. A major schism persists between critics and proponents of CAM – a schism that largely settles on the issue of evidence.

Patient use of CAM in theoretical context

As outlined in the Introduction, over the last two decades sociologists have engaged in debates about the implications of increased pluralism in healthcare, and indeed, the character of different forms of practice, evidence and knowledge production. Sociological research on CAM has drawn on a range of theoretical traditions to conceptualise developments, with numerous attempts made at linking CAM use to a societal shift to 'postmodernity'; processes of reflexive modernisation; and the emergence of new forms of 'selfhood'. As we shall illustrate, these conceptual arguments have often been speculatively linked to grand theory with little grounding in empirical data.

The postmodernisation thesis has been deployed as an explanation for the increased presence of CAM. Postmodernity denotes a transformation in social, cultural, economic and political arrangements, including differentiation, aestheticisation and the fragmentation of experience, with multiple ways of experiencing space and time (Cahoone, 1996). Postmodernism, however, is a cultural environment characterised by a pastiche of cultural styles and elements, implying a scepticism regarding order and progress, and promoting diversity and fragmentation. Proponents of the postmodernisation thesis view CAM use as reflecting wider patterns related to the 'postmodernisation' of social life (see Introduction for further discussion). Implicit in such arguments is the increased prioritisation of lay knowledges of disease and, importantly, a rejection of the superiority of scientific knowledge and expertise. While this theory has been widely drawn on, its applicability has been seriously questioned and has rarely been subject to empirical investigation (Tovey *et al.*, 2001).

Social theorisations of late modernity have also been drawn on in attempts to conceptualise patients' preferences for CAM (Low, 2004; Tovey *et al.*, 2001). Moving beyond the rather oversimplistic 'fragmentation of experience' and 'individualisation' themes implicit in the postmodernisation thesis, authors like Beck (1992) and Giddens (1991) have focused on increased reflexivity in modern societies and the tendency of 'consumers' to be more critical of expert knowledges. The result, it has been argued, is that people have become more sceptical of the judgements or advice of (scientific) experts (Lupton and Tulloch, 2002), actively assessing the merits of particular claims. This, in turn, it has been postulated, has opened up the potential for the proliferation of CAM – a backlash against the perceived failings of science and biomedical technologies (Kaptchuk and Eisenberg, 1998).

There have also been very recent attempts to theorise the potential implications, at an individual level, of new therapeutic models of care and their implications for changing notions of selfhood (e.g. Doel and Segrott, 2003; Sointu, 2006; Wray, 2007). This work has examined the degree to which CAM use represents a significant shift in conceptions of disease and selfhood. In particular, the notion of *wellbeing* has emerged recently as a potentially useful concept for characterising what CAM offers to the individual. Departing from biomedical notions of being 'cured', 'healthy' or 'disease free', *wellbeing* encapsulates notions of authenticity, recognition and self-determination; restructuring 'health' as a subjective and individualised process (Bishop and Yardley, 2004; Sointu, 2006; Wray, 2007). CAM use is thus conceptualised as a project of the self – an individual search for recognition as an authentic self that is both 'discovered' by the individual and shaped by the nature of individual therapeutic practices. Social theorisations of *wellbeing* have emphasised the limitations of biomedical conceptions of disease and health, and are thus, in part, a natural conceptual extension of the depersonalisation (e.g. McClean, 2005) and deindividualisation (e.g. Anspach, 1988) theses. These two latter arguments refer broadly to processes by which many biomedical clinicians abstract from the individual through speech (i.e. referring to 'the patient'), technologies (i.e. the person as a biomedicalised image), statistical probabilities (i.e. the group rather than individual), units of analysis (e.g. genes/cellular) and so on, rather than acknowledging the individual subject. This is seen to alienate the patient from treatment processes – perhaps even resulting in the need for alternative therapeutic options.

As illustrated above, and in the Introduction, sociological theory as applied to CAM has tended to engage in the reification of broader socio-cultural shifts in relation to individual choice, conceptions of disease and lay/expert relations. Rather than reflecting broad paradigmatic change, we argue, based on the patient accounts presented below, that the increasing presence of CAM in cancer care should be characterised as a dialectical tension between therapeutic processes engendering individuation (e.g. agency/self-responsibility/wellbeing/individual healing) and depersonalisation (e.g. cure rates/probabilities/abstraction). Moreover, the ways in which patients attempt to manage this dialectic are deeply embedded in the nature of their disease (i.e. disease stage and prognosis) and age.

Cancer patients' perspectives on scientific evidence

A central issue for this study was to achieve an understanding of the ways these cancer patients view scientific evidence and the conceptual basis of their assessments of the legitimacy of scientific knowledge in decision-making. Participants' responses were quite varied. However, what was clear was that a significant number of these patients viewed 'evidence' and 'scientific' knowledge as highly problematic concepts. Moreover, their views regarding the nature of 'evidence production' were often closely interlinked with their use of non-biomedical treatments:

PARTICIPANT: It is very difficult to get any information on [ovarian cancer] apart from statistics and how many folk die with [ovarian cancer] and that wasn't what I wanted, that wasn't what I needed . . . I mean, they [doctors] are not God, they don't know how long somebody has got to live, I don't care who they are . . . Some people get given a prognosis and they will live. The statistics take away something if you listen to them. They take away hope . . . your own ability to heal yourself.

(female, 58 years, ovarian, metastatic)

Another respondent:

INTERVIEWER: How important is scientific evidence for you?
PARTICIPANT: Not particularly. I don't think so, because, as medicine itself is an interaction between the individual and what you are giving them . . . So, you could take 100 people and it might not work for 70 of them, but if they are not working with it, that is why it is not working . . . also, you personally haven't got a 70 per cent chance of cure anyway. It's that 70 per cent of people will be cured, that's different isn't it?

(female, 51 years, bowel, metastatic)

Another respondent:

PARTICIPANT: Science can only take you so far. I'm a religious person so I'm quite spiritual so there's all that side of things and there's evidence from your own experience which you may not be able to write down in a formula. So, I mean . . . I don't care; it's not the be all and end all what science says, although I respect it.

(female, 70 years, ovarian, metastatic)

Another respondent:

PARTICIPANT: I have been to see a very eminent healer called [name of healer] who is a wonderful man in [name of location] and I have healing sessions from him and my first healing session last year with him I ended up in horrendous pain for two days. There was such a shift in my body, it's like surgery on the inside and then I felt wonderful after that. Now to the non-believer it sounds like hocus pocus but I don't care, I don't give a dam, it makes me feel better. I don't need scientific studies to tell me, I don't need these double-blind random studies. They make me feel well and balanced and back in control able to fight the disease as best I can. I know when there's time to go and nobody, no doctor, no healer . . . my healer's wife died of cancer last February, there was nothing he could do but that's the time to go, it's your time to go and I would like to go peacefully. I am not in denial, I am not running away from my cancer, but I'd just like to be in control, informed about the treatments, and I feel that the alternative treatments I have help me stay in control, give me a boost, make me feel strong, make me feel well. I have reflexology; I have just had a session this morning.

(female, 48 years, breast cancer, advanced)

As illustrated above, a significant proportion of these patients, regardless of whether they had opted to use CAMs or not, had ambivalent (if not negative) feelings towards statistics and probabilities on 'cure'. Given the fact that most were still undergoing treatment, whether for potentially curable or metastatic disease, they were faced with the difficult task of trying to decide who to trust. Moreover, they each attempted critically to assess the paradigmatic basis of the knowledge that was being given to them, often coming up with complex critiques of different forms of knowledge. Biomedicine was not, in large part, considered flawed as a discipline, nor were statistics viewed as having no use. In fact, most of these patients acknowledged that statistics were accurate in terms of how the *average number* of people will react to a particular treatment. However, a significant proportion felt that this told them little about how they personally would react to treatment. Lifestyle, emotion and spirituality were often described as factors that may heavily influence whether you were, for example, in the 70 per cent who were 'cured' or the 30 per cent who were not.

As illustrated in the second excerpt shown above, a common view was that it was not that one had a certain percentage chance of survival, but, rather, that a certain percentage of people would survive. Initially this seems like splitting hairs, but in fact it vividly illustrates what many participants felt biomedical statistics could not give them – concrete knowledge about how they, a unique individual, would react to treatment. Statistics were viewed as a crude conglomerate of disparate bodies and unique lives. Thus, although biomedical evidence was viewed as able accurately to show effectiveness over the wider patient population, it was not viewed as able to show the effectiveness of a treatment for a specific individual.

As is shown later, this logic was also crucial in terms of decisions to utilise CAM. For some, their experience of biomedical decision-making processes led them to develop a critical view of medical statistics and to seek out and use CAMs. For others, critiques of biomedical knowledge had been learnt from their CAM practitioner/s and were deployed to justify their decision-making in relation to biomedicine (or their rejection of their prognosis). In such cases, CAM therapists had employed ideological critiques of biomedical statistics to justify the lack of 'evidence' to back up their own treatments and the individual patient would utilise this framework to make sense of the legitimacy of the CAM therapy and the restrictive nature of their prognosis.

It is important to emphasise that patients' views of evidence were embedded in, but not dictated by, the nature of their disease (stage and prognosis). It was acknowledged by several of the patients that the better the statistical probability of cure, regardless of the flaws inherent in the application of statistics to the individual, the less likely it was to be a bad result for the individual. Thus, their critiques of biomedical statistics, perhaps unsurprisingly, were very much linked to feelings of ambiguity about the result:

PARTICIPANT: One is hardly going to argue about cure rates when faced with a 90 per cent chance of cure. You'd say, 'Thank God for that.' You really only start to question statistics when they aren't going your way. Or, I suppose, when it [the treatment outcome] could go either way. Also, what they say [CAM therapists] is also going to be more appealing I suppose.

Later in the interview:

PARTICIPANT: I must say, I am more critical [of science] now than earlier [before treatment]. Of course I thought the result would be a lot better than it was.

(female, 45 years, breast, metastatic)

In certain situations, impressive success rates require little consideration of other factors that may play a role in healing or, indeed, enlisting alternative models of healing. This was illustrated in the accounts of some of the patients with localised tumours or curable metastatic disease who were told they had an excellent chance of cure. Thus, patients' perceptions of and tendency to critically assess biomedical evidence were very much embedded in the 'odds' they were given and how acceptable they felt these were. The more ambiguous or negative the 'odds' were, the more statistics were viewed as unable to predict outcomes. Moreover, the degree to which the prognosis was acceptable seemed to be mediated by age.

Whereas the younger patients tended to have real difficulty accepting their prognosis, older patients often experienced fewer problems accepting a prognosis of around, say, a five-year survival. As one 73-year-old male with prostate cancer said, 'I've had a pretty good run so far so I'm not bothered really.' In such cases, patients were less likely to question prognostic data, use whole-system CAMs or develop critiques of biomedical knowledge. This, it would seem, may also be connected to (potentially hegemonic) discourses of ageing and perceptions of coming to a 'natural end' rather than the need to 'fight' and 'get well':

PARTICIPANT: I was very interested in my son's cancer . . . I really wanted to know all about that but I never really cared about [my cancer] and finding out information. I thought, I'm older, this is my lot. I mean he's younger; it was a big tragedy you know.

(female, 70 years, ovarian, metastatic)

Thus, it may the case that the need to challenge one's prognosis and question evidence (and in fact potentially utilise CAMs) may be embedded in wider cultural constructions of the appropriateness of 'sickness' or indeed 'cure' for certain age groups and types of individuals. In saying this, as is illustrated later in this discussion, the younger cancer patients interviewed here have grown up in the context of a *relative* waning in deference to biomedical expertise. Thus, these intersecting but also distinct factors (i.e. age and medico-cultural context) potentially mediate these patients' perceptions of evidence and CAM as well as their tendency to accept or question their actual prognosis.

It also emerged from the interviews that 'what is rational' is very much situated, in that when faced with a terminal illness people will question established knowledge that otherwise they would not. This was not viewed as an act of desperation, but critical thinking at a pivotal point in life:

PARTICIPANT: These people that sit there saying, 'How do you believe in these therapies?' They are not where we are. Have any of these people got terminal cancer or a terminal disease? They aren't in that position, so they don't know, it's like anything, as much as you commiserate, you do not really fully understand what it's like . . . you have got to be in that position to fully understand how it feels . . . and if you were in this position, you'd get out there and try things.

(female, 58 years, ovarian, metastatic)

Another respondent:

INTERVIEWER: As your prognosis changed, did your need for complementary therapies?
PARTICIPANT: I think, yes, obviously I have moved more that way now because they [medical specialists] are not offering me much anymore, so I am prepared to give it a go . . . and you question whether what they say [medical specialists] is really true.

(female, 51 years, bowel, advanced)

These patients' critiques of science, biomedical knowledge and utilisation of CAMs, in this context, could be construed as a response to the uncertainty of an ambiguous diagnosis, and indeed these patients were fully aware of this discourse of CAM use. As illustrated in the second excerpt above, some of these patients recall making a deliberate decision to investigate non-biomedical options and question biomedical statistics as their prognosis worsened, an illustration of how perceptions evolve over the disease process. However, although fear and uncertainty undoubtedly contribute to perceptions of scientific evidence and alternative models of care, decision-making processes are much more complex and cannot be reduced to a need for hope in the face of death. Rather, critiques of depersonalisation and abstraction, and value placed on the attributes of alternative forms (and models of) cancer care, need to be placed in the wider context of the need for subjectivity, agency and self-determination in disease and treatment processes.

Agency, subjectivity and self-determination

Participants' critiques of biomedical evidence tended to espouse a highly individualised view of disease and treatment response. Their reflections were sometimes drawn from their interactions with CAM practitioners, whereas for other patients they were the product of working through their emotions in relation to medical statistics and interactions with biomedical clinicians. Regardless of the origin of the critique, such feelings were characterised by a strong desire on the part of patients to retain their own subjectivity and self-determination. Statistics, in many cases, were seen to demoralise and take away 'hope'.

Scientific evidence and biomedical treatment processes were seen to limit human agency, produce anxiety and, in extreme cases, even induce death as patients choose to 'give up on life'. The imposition of the collective on the individual (or depersonalisation) was viewed, in such cases, as an unethical and ultimately counterproductive practice employed by many biomedical clinicians. In response to the threat of statistics on 'cure' rates, a number of the patients (although a distinct minority) refused to be told their prognosis. Although, in part, this was probably also about not wanting to hear potentially 'bad news', probability was seen to impose abstracted and oversimplified patterns on a subjective and unique individual (McClean, 2005).

For significant numbers of the patients with metastatic disease, their CAM practitioners often played a pivotal role in ensuring they had 'hope' and in countering the feelings of despondency resulting from their prognosis. Patients would develop a critique of biomedical evidence from conversations with their individual practitioner about the prognosis, a process that could be construed as CAM practitioners leading patients away from legitimate biomedical knowledge. However, if we look closer we see that patients place a high value on certain facets of alternative approaches to treatment – a value that cannot be reduced to a 'desperate' need for hope when faced by a negative prognosis:

INTERVIEWER: For you, in deciding whether to use a treatment or not, how important is the existence of scientific evidence?

PARTICIPANT: Quite important, although when I first started to see [CAM practitioner] and I spoke to other people about it, they always put an emphasis on what his results were like – the percentage of success rate. So often I ask [name of CAM practitioner] and he would say, 'Patients that I cure is 100 per cent success rate, patients that I don't is a 0 per cent success rate.' That would annoy me a bit because, well, that's not an answer, but what I realised is, how can he have these statistics, you have to look at cases, individual cases, you can't just put a figure at the end of it – a 70 per cent success rate.

(male, 25 years, LP nodular Hodgkins, metastatic)

Another respondent:

INTERVIEWER: How important is scientific evidence for you?

PARTICIPANT: Well, if [patients] are not working with [the treatment], that is why it is not working. It's not the therapy that is not working; it's the interaction between the individual and the therapy that is not working. Medical studies are always done at arm's length, so really your interaction with the people who are giving you the medicine is not considered, it's just irrelevant. So I think the evidence is whether it works for you.

(female, 51 years, bowel, metastatic)

Another respondent:

PARTICIPANT: I just think, no, sorry, you might not be able to equate it [CAM therapy]; you may not be able to put any sort of balance on it and say that it is researchable, quantifiable or whatever, but, yes, I just believe it works.

(female, 40 years, adrenal, metastatic)

Another respondent:

PARTICIPANT: I know this sounds odd but I feel I am quite scathing and sceptical about a lot of scientific methods . . . a lot of it to me seems to be barking up the wrong tree, so I don't go a whole bunch on evidence really. If somebody says to me, well, a friend of mine had lymphoma and she found that this was particularly helpful, something was particular helpful, I would prick my ears up and investigate it. But it would really matter to me how I felt about it because I do realise that everybody's story is different, and, you know, just like everybody's pregnancy is different, you can never say that if you go down the same route you will get the same result. Evidence to me is not as important.

(female, 45 years, lymphoma, metastatic)

Again we see how these patients, and many of the others interviewed, conceptualised 'evidence' in relation to CAM. It was not that they rejected outright the ability of statistics to tell them useful things about the successes of biomedical and CAM cancer treatments for a group; it is that science was not perceived to be able to predict what would happen to *them*, and to *their* body.

As we see in the first excerpt, such critiques of statistics and scientisation were often encouraged by their CAM practitioners, who also drew on highly individualised understandings of illness and the body. We see this again in the following description of a spiritual healer's approach:

PARTICIPANT: She reckoned the reason which I had got cancer, was because my chakras were not working . . . it was about a lack of energy balance in my body . . . It's totally different to the way doctors work . . . they [CAM practitioners] focus on *your* [emphasis] life and your individual stuff and not just the disease and statistics.

(male, 27 years, testicular, post-curative)

As a discipline, clinical epidemiology emerged as a method of ensuring that the clinician and the patient have a high degree of certainty about the effects of an intervention – all things being equal, processes of randomisation are designed to produce accurate chances of treatment success. As suggested by a number of the patients interviewed here, this very process of randomisation and abstraction may also obscure the impact of the individual on his/her body and disease.

The discourse of individuality is complicated by the fact that often these patients genuinely desired statistics to defend their use of a particular CAM practitioner to family and friends. At the same time, critiques of evidence were appealing given the fact that they appreciated the highly subjective nature of the treatment process and the importance of the individual in shaping the treatment outcome. In this sense, we have a complex combination of a prognosis, a desire for cure, but also a need for a paradigm which gives hope and a sense of control over one's fate.

It is important to note that the characteristics of the CAMs being used also potentially shapes patients' perspectives on evidence and biomedical care. Some of the practices used by these patients can be characterised as 'whole-systems' approaches like herbalism, homeopathy or naturopathy. Whereas these therapeutic systems seek to 'treat' the patient's cancer or symptomatology, other CAM practices such as healing touch or reiki may merely seek to alleviate pain or psychological distress. The latter practices also tend to involve limited discussion of ideology, whereas in the case of the whole-systems approaches, discussion of the paradigmatic basis of the treatment can be both a crucial part of the client/practitioner encounter and play a central role in shaping patients' perspectives on biomedical cancer care. As one patient recalled of her spiritual healer:

PARTICIPANT: She said not to worry about why it works but to let it work. She said she just helps the conventional treatments do their job and that's all. She made no claims to cure or anything . . . I don't think she liked that I had been told there was no hope for me but . . . she wasn't going to push me away from [doctors] . . . she wouldn't criticise them either.

> (female, age unknown, breast, metastatic)

Thus, we can see that the character of individual CAM users and the CAMs they utilise each potentially influence the propensity to critique scientific knowledge and biomedical prognoses.

Experiential knowledge, CAM therapies and trust in science

Dissatisfaction with biomedical science and statistics on cure rates often led these patients to try things out and pursue a trajectory whereby they would judge a treatment purely on the outcome rather than its philosophy or available statistical evidence. In some cases, patients had already used the particular type of CAM previously for a minor illness (e.g. homeopathic or herbal remedies), but most of the time patients merely tried out treatments they had heard of before but had never actually used. One patient described this process as a 'leap of faith' whereby the patient largely ignores the 'logic' behind the treatment:

PARTICIPANT: The things that I could see, I could see with healing, I could see physically that it was working. I could see that with the trances and the physical reactions that she [spiritual healer] was having in the room. So you couldn't prove that scientifically but I knew it was working. And the thing is, when she sort of recommended the crystals, because I knew the other things were working, I sort of went along with it really. I didn't understand scientifically how the crystals actually worked and . . . I wasn't really interested.

Later in the interview:

INTERVIEWER: How do you then decide if something, I mean if you haven't got evidence that something works in the sense of statistics, how on earth do you decide whether something is going to work?

PARTICIPANT: That's quite a difficult question to answer, but, you have feelings about things, they make sense to you. I presume that's why I think they will work. I mean, the stuff that I have been given is backed up enough with examples of other patients to make me think, well, yes, that will work for me . . .

INTERVIEWER: How do you pick out the good from the bad?

PARTICIPANT: I guess, first come first served.

INTERVIEWER: Try it out and see what happens?

PARTICIPANT: Yes, and then if something comes along and that sounds a bit better, then you might deviate.

(male, 25 years, LP nodular Hodgkins, metastatic)

Another patient:

PARTICIPANT: I have been [to the psychic surgeon] four times now . . . I read up about him on the Internet.

INTERVIEWER: Can you tell me what actually happened?

PARTICIPANT: Well, when you go, you don't say an awful lot. You don't have to say an awful lot. He feels for hot spots around your body that need surgery . . . the last time I went to see him he did surgery on my lungs. He used surgical instruments without the knives and sort of almost like pulls away at your body and pulls things out of your body, very strange experience.

INTERVIEWER: He uses surgical instruments in what sense?

PARTICIPANT: In terms of a scalpel handle [without the blade] . . . it is pretty uncomfy and he makes your skin red. He has never left any scars but it has taken a day or two days for that redness to go. [I was] sceptical initially . . . but last time I went he hit my lungs and he just did healing on my lungs. I didn't say anything but he did actually locate them [the tumours] . . . I was quite convinced by that.

(female, 40 years, adrenal, advanced)

Another respondent:

PARTICIPANT: I saw [the psychic surgeon] on telly years ago and I remembered his name, so I knew he had been doing it along time . . . you see him for three or four minutes and it's not a consultation by any means. He swans in, says 'Hi' to you, asks you how you are doing, cracks a couple of jokes, hands on, straight in, does this kind of imaginary surgery and he kind of just touches you and puts his hands in. And the first time I went I heard all this slopping. It was like a rummaging feeling but he is so quick, he says 'Hi' and he's in already and he has thrown stuff out and that's it finished.

INTERVIEWER: Throwing stuff out . . . like in the air . . .?

PARTICIPANT: He does this kind of thing and throwing kind of stuff, it's all energy stuff but its fascinating and then when I got up from there and I felt quite painful and when I got up from there it was painful. It was painful for about 12 hours I suppose and I had quite a big line across where he did it, it was quite sore. Anyway he doesn't offer an opinion, in fact I think one time [friend's name] asked him how she was doing and he said, 'Only God knows how you are doing. I don't know how you are doing.' So it doesn't profess to give you advice about your future or anything except he says you should live every moment as if it is your last really. Anyway I still do go to him . . . he works on my energy, my energy fields really and I think he can see and operate at a deep level which is not physical. So I think he is kind of one of my important members of my team because I don't think that you can, well, I don't think I can be healed just from a spiritual angle or just from a physical angle and I think there is a whole spectrum of things.

INTERVIEWER: How do you decide whether something is worth trying or not or something is effective?

PARTICIPANT: Sometimes it's what I hear about it, but, mostly, the most important thing to me is how it feels with me, if it feels right. I don't mean the things itself but the thought of doing that and being involved in it and I think it has to be something that resonates with me. There are certain things I wouldn't like to try.

(female, 45 years, lymphoma, Metastatic)

What emerged was a significant group of cancer patients prioritising experiential knowledge and rejecting the need for scientific evidence in treatment decisions. Some of the CAMs used, including spiritual healing and psychic surgery, involved what some would consider quite exotic practices, but yet these patients chose to judge the therapies on their effect rather than the basis of the practice itself. For many respondents, the 'science' behind the treatments was irrelevant and feeling 'better in myself' was the ultimate measure of whether a treatment was working or not.

The prioritising of experiential knowledge and scepticism toward science seemed closely linked to various historical events which were perceived to reflect the dangers of trusting 'expert' opinion and 'scientific' knowledge. Moreover, the willingness to experiment and try 'alternatives' was shown in the interviews to be embedded in a wider socio-historical context of waning trust in scientific expertise:

INTERVIEWER: To you, how important is scientific evidence.

PARTICIPANT: Not really, it's not important whatsoever. I'm now 57 and I see that many experts come out with so many wonderful ideas and then a few years later it comes as how it's a total load of rubbish . . . like the big thing about GM [genetically modified] foods, is it good or is it no good? If somebody in a white coat was to tell me something I wouldn't take it as God's gospel . . . I just try it and see if it works for me.

(male, 57 years, bowel, post-curative)

A number of patients felt that their ability to trust medical experts had been eroded by various medical controversies and perceived misinformation given to the public over the dangers of particular drugs and diseases. Thalidomide, genetically modified food and mad cow disease were often used as examples of the fallibility of medical advice and the need to make one's own assessments of both risk and benefit.

However, views of evidence and scientific knowledge were not linear. In fact, some patients rejected all forms of knowledge that did not draw on scientific method. As perhaps could be expected, these tended to be the non-CAM users in the study, although we should emphasise that CAM use was not a determining factor:

PARTICIPANT: I would never dream of giving up conventional medicine and my drugs. And, whatever they [the doctors] say to me, I do. Whatever they [doctors] say. If they say go and sit in a hot bath for three hours, I'd go and sit in a hot bath because I believe what they say. That's normal, I mean, why would you not?

(female, 69 years, uterus, metastatic)

Another respondent:

PARTICIPANT: I am a bit wary . . . I have read about things like the Gerson diet, and, I mean, they don't work. They die these people and to do something that is so radical without the proof that it works . . . no! [exclamation]. I need proof.

(female, 53 years, leukaemia, metastatic)

Another respondent:

PARTICIPANT: I will try things because I'm interested, you know, I just venture to so I'd heard about [a particular CAM practitioner]. In fact one of my chemo nurses knew her as well and said, 'Why don't you try [therapist's name]?' So I went down and I just . . . I found the room she had quite oppressive and bit kind of, not spooky, but a bit too mystical for me. Not clinical. And also I found her a bit patronising, you know, the way that she talked and the way that she was, as if . . . and I wondered if it's how people when they go to the hypnotist, you felt that a lot of the power was with the therapist and I felt, you know, like, 'Let me take it all away for you. Just relax and you'll be alright.' So I thought, 'This isn't for me,' which is fine, you know, and if some other people get something out of it, do it, you know. So I thought I'd tried it and I didn't want to try it a second time. I thought, well, you know, it wasn't for me.

(female, 50 years, breast, metastatic)

Although a minority in the overall sample, there were a number of patients who gave full support to the superiority of scientific knowledge. For these patients it was a matter of unconditional trust, in the sense that they would do absolutely anything their specialist told them to do. From this perspective, biomedicine had the best track record of success, the most rigorous research methods and was most ethical in its claims-making. Thus, we see a spectrum of views of 'evidence' and the legitimacy of biomedical knowledge within this study, emphasising the importance of a policy trajectory that also acknowledges significant differentiation in patients' views of, and desire for, a biomedical-type evidence base.

Discussion

In this chapter we have presented an empirical and conceptual examination of the ways in which NHS cancer patients conceptualise and utilise different forms of evidence in relation to CAM and biomedicine. We have illustrated that what CAM achieves for individual patients is not linear and patients' perceptions of and utilisation of different forms of evidence (scientific or otherwise) vary considerably according to the individual patient's ontological and epistemological positioning (which are in turn mediated by their disease and treatment trajectories).

Alternative models of healing were valued, primarily, for their subjectified (rather than abstracted) and individualised (rather than depersonalised) approach to cancer care; an approach that was seen to allow for, and promote, agency, self-determination and ultimately hope. CAM practitioners were seen by many of those interviewed to promote a 'project of the self'; a reclaiming of hope, subjectivity and control – elements that were largely perceived as neglected in biomedical cancer care (see Chapter 5 for how experiences can change over time). Particularly in cases of uncertainty and ambiguity about success rates, statistical probabilities were perceived to create an environment of determinism that promoted fatalism. There was not a rejection of the value of biomedical statistics but, rather, a critical view which emphasised their limited scope and weakness in predicting outcomes for the individual patient.

Cancer represents a highly specific context in which the consumption of CAM has particular meanings (and serves particular roles), meanings that may be very different from those observed in other disease and health contexts. The threat of terminal illness clearly has considerable implications for patients' preparedness to go beyond traditional notions of evidence and effectiveness; moreover, therapeutic approaches that promote indeterminacy ('my fate is unclear') and self-determination ('I can make a difference') are going to be extremely appealing to many patients who have metastatic or advanced disease.

Ultimately most of the patients interviewed here still considered biomedical knowledge and expertise as playing an important role in their cancer care, regardless of the difficulties they had with evidence and statistical probabilities. Thus, at least within this context, conceptually, the notions of a broader paradigm shift (postmodernity), increasing distrust in science (reflexive modernisation) or the emergence of a forms of identity work (individual wellbeing), alone, do not capture the complexity of these patients' engagement with CAM and biomedicine. Although these conceptual arguments each provide some insight into what is a complex social phenomenon, what characterises these patients' engagement with CAM in cancer care is a complex dialectical tension between the appeal of individualisation (recognition of the subjective self) and depersonalisation (appeal of control and certainty) – a tension that for most patients is not actually resolved but rather managed through the disease and treatment processes.

The management of this dialectic – or indeed the appeal of these ontological extremes – was shown in this study to be inextricably tied to these patients' own desire for (and thus the attraction of) particular ontological and epistemological positions within the management of their specific disease. Thus, we advocate a theoretical approach that acknowledges both the emerging dialectic between individuation and depersonalisation, but also the role of physiological and demographic factors (e.g. age) which influence how individual patients attempt to resolve such tensions.

Conclusion

UK cancer policy in relation to CAM is in its infancy, and that which does exist is largely directed by a need for a biomedical-type evidence base. This current policy trajectory does not acknowledge the kinds of ontological and epistemological complexities that the cancer patients interviewed here engage with, such as: what constitutes 'evidence' for me, in my life; does abstract biomedical knowledge apply to the individual; and exactly who (and what) decides what constitutes legitimate knowledge of disease and treatment processes? As illustrated in these patients' accounts, decision-making about CAM is mediated by a range of complex personal and social processes and 'scientific' evidence may or may not play an influential role in decision-making. This is largely a reflection of the fact that many cancer patients seem acutely aware of the contingent and ultimately multifaceted nature of evidence and knowledge of the body.

We argue, therefore, that the production of a biomedical-type evidence base for CAM may not actually have a significant influence on cancer patients' decisions to use CAM or on their views of it. Policy must reflect the types of complex issues that cancer patients face in decision-making and treatment processes including the multifaceted nature of notions such as 'evidence' and 'effectiveness'.

2 The role of the Internet in cancer patients' engagement with therapeutic options

Introduction

Health information has proliferated via the Internet over the last decade and patients are increasingly able to access a multitude of biomedical and non-biomedical knowledges about health, illness and the body. Studies are now showing that patients, and cancer patients in particular, regularly use the Internet to collect information and make treatment decisions (e.g. Chen and Siu, 2001). As a result, medical sociologists have, in recent years, examined the significance and impact of the Internet within the context of healthcare, resulting in a considerable body of work addressing the potential implications for patients, clinicians and the structure of healthcare delivery (e.g. Anderson *et al.*, 2003; Broom, 2005; Broom, 2005a; Burrows *et al.*, 2000; Hardey, 1999, 2002; Nettleton *et al.*, 2005; Seale, 2005; Sharf, 1997; Ziebland, 2004; Ziebland *et al.*, 2004). However, hitherto there has been no sociological research examining the impact of the Internet within the context of cancer patients' utilisation of complementary and alternative medicine (CAM).

This is despite the fact that, particularly in the case of cancer, the Internet is often represented as problematic, or even harmful (see Schmidt and Ernst, 2004), because of its so-called tendency to sway patients away from biomedical cancer treatments or mislead them in relation to their side-effects (Kiley, 2002; McKinley *et al.*, 1999; Whiting, 2000). Moreover, over the last decade there has been significant conjecture from biomedical clinicians and researchers as to the role of the Internet as a porthole to inaccurate information or so-called 'unproven' treatments (Cline and Haynes, 2001; S. Fox, 2005; Ernst and Schmidt, 2002; Schmidt and Ernst, 2004). Some social commentators have reinforced such representations by conceptualising the Internet as having so-called 'democratising effects', and promoting therapeutic pluralism (Goldstein, 2004), in a socio-cultural context hitherto dominated by a biomedical view of illness (e.g. N. Fox *et al.*, 2005; Hardey, 1999, 2002). However, thus far no data has been provided to substantiate such arguments, and indeed there is emerging criticism of the liberative or emancipatory potential of information technologies more broadly (e.g. Agre, 2002) and in the specific context of healthcare (e.g. Broom, 2005; Henwood *et al.*, 2003).

The aim of this chapter is to examine the role of the Internet in cancer patients' engagement with CAM. In doing this we argue: (1) that previous representations of the Internet as a porthole to CAM are oversimplistic and that access to biomedical knowledge may pose far greater problems to patients (particularly those who are CAM users); and (2) that social theorisations of the Internet should be revisited to examine potential limitations in their application to the context of cancer.

Background

Sociological studies of the Internet in healthcare have examined different facets of its influence, including its implications for expert knowledge (N. Fox *et al.*, 2005; Hardey, 1999); the doctor/patient relationship (Broom, 2005; Anderson *et al.*, 2003; Henwood *et al.*, 2003); patients' treatment choices; patient/patient interactions (Broom, 2005b; Sharf, 1997); patients' experience of disease (Broom, 2005a; Nettleton and Burrows, 2003; Seale *et al.*, 2006; Ziebland, 2004; Ziebland *et al.*, 2004); and health policy (Burrows *et al.*, 2000). This wealth of sociological research has illustrated the strong influence of new information technologies (and forms of online interaction) within healthcare delivery (see also Cotton, 2001).

However, hitherto there has been no research into the role of the Internet in cancer patients' usage of and perceptions of CAM. This is despite the fact that medical associations and biomedical clinicians and researchers themselves regularly blame the Internet for the proliferation of complementary and alternative medicines (e.g. FTC, 2001) or hold it responsible for pushing some patients away from biomedical cancer treatments (e.g. Ernst and Schmidt, 2002; Kiley, 2002; Whiting, 2000). It is common, for example, in the UK to see media reports representing cancer patients as being 'ripped off' by online quackery – a typical construction being the vulnerable cancer patient who is desperate for a cure for their disease (e.g. Ernst and Schmidt, 2002; Jarvis, 2005). Regardless of such claims, little is known about why patients may or may not use the Internet as a means of accessing CAM. Moreover, the existence of biomedical diagnostic and prognostic information online is often presented as unproblematic despite the possibility that patients' accessing of *biomedical* information may in fact have considerable emotional and psychological implications. Moreover, and particularly in the context of the patients interviewed here, in a medico-cultural context where patients are increasingly pursuing alternative trajectories in their cancer treatment, what is 'fact' or 'evidence' can be highly contingent (Broom and Tovey, 2007a), thus problematising simplistic conceptions of 'misinformation' or 'quackery' online.

Internet use by cancer patients and CAM

The limited research that has been done suggests that Internet use is variable amongst cancer patients (e.g. Lea *et al.*, 2005). Eysenbach (2003) reported that of 24 identified surveys that contain data on the proportion of persons with cancer who are Internet users, the average proportion of Internet users is 39 per cent (ranging from 4 per cent to 58 per cent). In their study Chen and Siu (2001) found that 16.7 per cent of patients estimated that they had spent between 10 and 30 hours, and 23.8 per cent spent more than 30 hours, searching for information about their cancer on the Internet. In this same study, 53.7 per cent of respondents reported that the information they received from their physicians and other healthcare providers was insufficient. Differences in Internet usage between patient groups have also been shown, with a study by Metz *et al.* (2003) illustrating significant differentiation according to cancer type: lung 16 per cent; head and neck 18 per cent; prostate 27 per cent; breast 34 per cent; and gynaecologic 45 per cent.

There has been virtually no work done on the Internet as a pathway to complementary and alternative medicine for cancer patients and none that is sociologically informed. Studies of the general population give some indication of the Internet as a pathway to CAM-related information. For example, a US study found that 30 per cent of Internet users search for information on 'alternative' therapies (S. Fox, 2005). Moreover, although there is only very limited quantitative data available at present, some reports suggest that the Internet may represent a pathway to CAM for certain patient groups (e.g. Eng *et al.*, 2003). However, such studies tell us little about *why* patients – and cancer patients in particular – search for certain kinds of information and how they view and utilise this information once they have retrieved it.

Social theory and the Internet

Theoretical debate around patients' experiences of the Internet has focused on experiences of empowerment and self-determination as patients are exposed to information about their healthcare and different therapeutic models of care (Broom, 2005; Hardey, 1999; Sharf, 1997). Analysis has tended to focus on the potentially liberating impact of the Internet for patients (Hardey, 1999, 2002; Radin, 2006) as well as the potential dangers posed by a so-called democratisation of health information online. The ease of access to a range of knowledges (and the ability to share experiences online) has led some commentators to the conclusion that the Internet has fundamentally empowered patients, promoting individual autonomy and agency in treatment and decision-making processes (Hardey, 1999; Pitts, 2004; Radin, 2006; Sharf, 1997).

Another major stream of social theory, as applied to the Internet, has developed in terms of the medical professional and, in particular, the degree to which the Internet challenges the traditional authority of the medical 'expert'. Argument has centred on the disruption of the 'expert's' exclusive access to knowledge (e.g. Anderson *et al.*, 2003; Diaz *et al.*, 2002; N. Fox and Roberts, 1999), and indeed its role in challenging the traditional asymmetric 'competence' that is at the heart of professional identity (see Hardey, 1999;

Ziebland, 2004). This has included theorisations of a diminution in public deference to expert knowledge (the reflexive possibility of late modernisation) and processes of deprofessionalisation (i.e. a demystification of expert knowledge) as seen in increased questioning of doctors' authority (Beck, 1992; Broom, 2005; Hardey, 1999; Haug, 1988). The Internet-informed patient has thus been conceptualised as a part of the wider departure from the traditional Parsonian sick role to a more consumer-orientated 'active' role whereby patients are able to question professional advice-giving; a process that can influence patient roles and clinical autonomy (albeit differentially according to class, education, etc.). Such arguments have been changed in recent years as sociologists begin to emphasise the often contradictory effects of the Internet for the lay/professional interface (e.g. Broom, 2005; Henwood *et al.*, 2003) and more general sociological work emphasising the importance of acknowledging complexity within organisational settings and intra-professional differentiation (e.g. Timmermans and Kolker, 2004).

There has also been some work done on the potential of the Internet to have a liberating or egalitarian effect and, in the context of healthcare, to contribute to a gradual democratisation of medical knowledge (e.g. Goldstein, 2004; Light, 2001). Notions of therapeutic pluralism (Goldstein, 2004) and ideological shifts in conceptions of the self (and of the body) have been theorised according to notions of wellbeing (e.g. Sointu, 2006; Wray, 2007) and the postmodernisation of contemporary therapeutic landscapes (e.g. Eastwood, 2000). Patient engagement with CAM, it has been argued, represents one aspect of a broader socio-cultural shift in values and conceptions of the self and the body. According to some social commentators, developments such as the Internet have facilitated, or at the very least contributed to, the emergence of these broader ideological shifts through acting as a porthole to non-biomedical knowledges and therapeutic practices (Coulter and Willis, 2004). However, the notion of a pluralistic development that would contest (and potentially transform) the dominance of biomedicine (or indeed, increased patient engagement with alternative therapeutics) has not been backed up by empirical data. In this study we aimed to examine the degree to which the above conceptualisations of the Internet have relevance in the context of cancer and CAM engagement.

The Internet, prognosis and despondency

As suggested above, the Internet has often been represented as potentially dangerous due to its potential role as a porthole to the 'unproven' (Diaz *et al.*, 2002; Kiley, 2002; Schmidt and Ernst, 2004; Stoll, 1995; Whiting, 2000). Despite this common perception, for the majority of the cancer patients interviewed here, their main concern regarding the Internet was not inaccurate information or 'false claims'; rather, it was exposure to biomedical information that created the most anxiety:

PARTICIPANT: I went on the Cancer Research [UK] website and I knew the chances of [cancer] coming back were equal to it not, so I was thinking, well, it's a 50/50 chance of it coming back that's fine. What I didn't realise was that there is a 50/50 chance of being alive in five years which is very different sort of statistic to face. I did have a major panic about it . . . it really did just add to the stress of the whole situation.

(female, Scottish, 29 years, malignant melanoma, metastatic)

Another respondent:

PARTICIPANT: After the initial consultation I had six weeks before they told me the results. So I had six weeks of waiting by a telephone, which was horrendous, and all the time I was thinking to myself, my God, it could be spreading all over my body . . . because I had the Internet, I was delving into all sorts of frightening information all the time . . . I didn't really know what I was looking for, I was going into ovarian cancer. The more I did that, the more scared I was, you know?

(female, English, 49 years, Myloma, Metastatic)

As illustrated in the above excerpts and in many of the other interviewees' accounts, the primary difficulty these cancer patients experienced with the Internet was accessing (and, if necessary, avoiding) biomedical diagnostic and prognostic information. An overwhelming response was that the Internet posed a significant threat to their emotional wellbeing in terms of exposure to negative prognostic *biomedical* information. Particularly for those with metastatic or advanced disease, the Internet presented more of an emotional risk than a useful method of research – a technology that would emphasise, at least through a biomedical lens, how little time they had left or indeed how serious their condition was. This was emphasised particularly in the case of the more aggressive and well-known cancers (e.g. ovarian or malignant melanoma), where it was 'common knowledge' that the probability of survival is relatively low (which increases the likelihood of one accessing such information):

PARTICIPANT: I think I'm glad I didn't look on the internet when I was diagnosed. [My husband] did and survival rates for ovarian cancer were very, very low because they don't ever get the symptoms. So I didn't know that, I didn't know how many people it killed . . . with breast cancer, you know . . . it's a nice easy one to get aware of, isn't it, because it's easily diagnosed. There's something you can do to look for it and if you do diagnose it early then there's, you know, a nice cure rate. So it's quite a positive thing to concentrate on, whereas ovarian cancer is a bit of a black hole. No one knows what causes it or how it happens. They can have an idea about how to treat it but they're not very successful if it's a late diagnosis and there are no symptoms . . . Seeing that [Internet] information early on would have devastated me.

(female, 28 years, ovarian, undergoing potentially curable treatment)

Not only were patient experiences differentiated according to cancer type, it was also evident that the Internet had quite specific effects depending on what point in the diagnostic, disease or treatment stage it was being used. In a significant proportion of the other interviews, high levels of anxiety were reported when searching on the Internet between the initial consultation (in which a biopsy was often done, which was then sent to pathology) and the actual diagnosis and/or prognosis. This anxiety seemed heightened for both those with less common cancers and those with the more aggressive cancers. In the case of the less common cancers (e.g. multiple myloma or pancreatic cancer), patients often have little idea of which websites to visit due to the paucity of sites available, and for the more aggressive cancers they may access data on very poor survival rates before they even know their actual disease stage and the aggressiveness of the malignancy (pancreatic cancer falls into both the former and the latter categories).

From these patients' accounts it seems evident that when there is a significant time period between the initial consultation and the diagnosis accessing the Internet may also be highly problematic, and indeed significant attention needs to be given to this issue by medical specialists (i.e. guidance about what to search for, what to avoid and the range of potential outcomes in terms of stage and aggressiveness). However, for those post-biomedical treatment and in remission or potentially cured, looking on the Internet for non-biomedical options (particularly diet or healing-based therapies) was at times useful.

Although for some of these patients negative biomedical prognostic information was merely an 'added stress', for others it was viewed as playing a much more problematic role in their experiences of disease and treatment processes – it was seen to interfere with their pursuit of alternative healing processes.

Non-biomedical therapeutic models and the bio-medicalisation of the Internet

For some cancer patients – and bear in mind that the patients here are largely CAM users – the Internet presents a real barrier to their individual illness and treatment trajectories. Despite previous representations of online pluralism, rather than encouraging and facilitating CAM use or increasing scepticism toward biomedical cancer care, the Internet was perceived by many here to problematise their ability to heal themselves through non-biomedical therapeutics. A process of potential (or actual) bio-medicalisation via the Internet was evident with a significant number frustrated with continually being reminded of their 'prognosis'; the restrictive effect of their 'diagnosis' for alternative healing practices; and the despondency that can emerge from hope being taken away. Such feelings were often characterised by a desire for a sense of self-determination (rather than a fixed prognosis) that would allow for a sense of individual agency and promote self-healing (see also Broom and Tovey, 2007a):

PARTICIPANT: Well, the Internet I have sourced for [information about] adrenal cancer initially, and the maximum anybody had lived with adrenal cancer is twelve years. Therefore, the information I got off that was just like straightaway negative. No thank you [spoken authoratively] I am not just living twelve years. I am living longer than that. So the Internet was a negative source . . . When I started to look into adrenal cancer [on the Internet] and then started out finding out the statistics it scared me off and it gave me a lack of positivity . . . it gave me such a negative outlook, it just gave me such a complete low that it didn't help me heal myself.

(female, English, 40 years, adrenal, metastatic)

Another respondent:

PARTICIPANT: It is very difficult to get any information on [ovarian cancer] apart from statistics and how many folk die with [ovarian cancer] and that wasn't what I wanted, that wasn't what I needed . . . the statistics take away something if you listen to them. They take away hope . . . your own ability to heal yourself.

(female, 58 years, ovarian, metastatic)

Many of these patients avoided ongoing use of the Internet for fear of exposure to biomedically defined 'cure rates' that, from their perspective, would hinder a potential 'healing' process. This was often closely linked with their use of alternative therapeutic models. The CAM journey, for many of these patients, meant limiting their exposure to biomedical prognostic information (and thus the Internet) as much as possible. Moreover, those who did access CAM information off the Internet were highly sceptical of claims to cure and tended to utilise multiple sources of validation (e.g. friends, nurses, doctors and other CAM therapists) to assess the veracity of claims presented online.

These findings cast significant doubt on previous conceptions of the Internet as playing an empowering role for cancer patients and, moreover, of its tendency toward facilitating a democratisation of knowledge, exposing patients to and promoting alternative therapeutic models. This is not to suggest, of course, that the presence of biomedicine online is purely negative. Rather, that assumptions about the Internet as intrinsically pluralistic and tending towards critiques of biomedicine (rather than its promotion) need to be reassessed.

Strategies to limit danger online

Contrary to the commonly held view of cancer patients as relatively uncritical of the Internet and the information they retrieve online (e.g. Gilliam *et al.*, 2003), the patients interviewed here who did access the Internet were highly selective regarding the websites they visited and the information they retrieved.

Patients tended to be suspicious of both CAM and biomedical information, often questioning the cure rates presented by biomedical experts but also the claims of CAM organisations. For most of the patients interviewed here, restricting the scope of their information-searching on the Internet was the key to minimising harm from inaccurate information. Moreover, the information retrieved, more often than not, served merely to remind them of information already provided by the medical specialist, specialist cancer nurse or complementary therapist:

PARTICIPANT: We didn't allow ourselves to go onto the Internet [that much] and search because it was dangerous. I could have ended up having anything and being close to death's door.

INTERVIEWER: So you didn't trust the Internet, as such, is that what you mean?

PARTICIPANT: No [I didn't]. I have merely used sort of the Cancer Research UK site, Bristol Cancer Centre site, those sort of things, really just to reinforce what I am already thinking and maybe just for a little bit more information about what homeopathy is in general and those sort of things. I have not used their information to make decisions.

(female, English, 31 years, non-Hodgkin's lymphoma, metastatic)

Another respondent:

PARTICIPANT: I think you have to be very cautious about things you see on the Internet because there's a lot of stuff which isn't accredited. So I would trust people like Cancer BACUP [UK cancer organisation], and like my lymphoma association, and accredited people like that, that have got good information. I wouldn't go on, say, this wonderful new therapy that everybody is raving about in America, because I don't think it would be sound. I like things that are tested.

(female, English, 63 years, myloma, metastatic)

As we see in the excerpts above, these patients, and many of the others interviewed, took a highly sceptical approach to seeking information on the Internet, only trusting institutionally affiliated sites and sometimes avoiding the Internet altogether. Again, this goes against the stereotype of the uncritical cancer patient erratically seeking information online. In actuality, it would seem, at least from these results, that cancer patients are highly selective about the information they retrieve online:

INTERVIEWER: Do you trust the internet?

PARTICIPANT: No, no, it's just information and you have to make it what you will.

INTERVIEWER: Who or what do you trust the most in terms of the sources of information about complementary therapies?

PARTICIPANT: I think people, you know, who have actually tried it are always interesting, and if they approve [long pause] I guess I think, 'Can I go on that?'

> (female, English, 58 years, breast, metastatic)

Another respondent:

PARTICIPANT: I am dreadfully cynical [of the Internet] and I look at it and think, 'Who the hell is that?' . . . I didn't feel some of the sites were any better than women's magazines.

> (female, English, 52 years, breast, received
> potentially curable treatment)

Another respondent:

PARTICIPANT: One thing which is extremely dangerous to my way of thinking is any information you might get off the Internet . . . they are all trying to sell you something and it's marvellous, you know, until it kills you off [laughs]. Everything is so marvellous and wonderful, you know. 'Have two of these. Oh yes, go on, take four.' [You have to] make absolutely certain that any information . . . is bonafide.

> (male, Italian, 69 years, prostate, metastatic, remission)

It emerged that very few patients trusted the Internet as a source of information or support, whether biomedical or non-biomedical. Patients were particularly concerned about not being able to judge the qualifications of the people making claims and not being able to judge the veracity of the claims of people trying to propagate CAM or biomedicine. Given the fact that the majority of these patients were CAM users, this finding is significant, in that it seems likely that these patients would be more open to websites proposing alternative paradigms of care than cancer patients who are non-CAM users. However, it would seem from these results that one cannot conflate use of CAM with acceptance of online CAM information. Rather, much like with other sources of information, patients are highly sceptical regarding claims-making.

Discussion

Previous sociological analysis of the Internet has focused heavily on its potential to disrupt existing monopolies over medical knowledge and medical work and, furthermore, potentially transform patients into experts about their own disease and treatment trajectories (Broom, 2005; Hardey, 1999, 2002; Sharf, 1997). Moreover, there has been much speculation, although little empirical investigation, into the role of the Internet in promoting alternative paradigms of care and contributing to increased therapeutic pluralism (Diaz *et al.*, 2002; Goldstein, 2004; Schmidt and Ernst, 2004). The Internet, conceptually, has been linked to processes of patient empowerment, democratisation and deprofessionalisation (e.g. Hardey, 1999); but yet the results presented here suggest that such arguments (at the very least) need reassessment in the context of cancer patients' engagement with CAM.

Rather than engendering a process of deprofessionalisation or the promotion of therapeutic pluralism (Dudley *et al.*, 1996; Goldstein, 2004; Hardey, 1999), these results suggest that the Internet may be complicit in processes of biomedicalisation that reinforce a mechanistic biomedical conception of cancer and, at least for some patients, may restrict engagement with non-biomedical therapeutics. Particularly for cancer patients who are CAM users, the Internet can be a form of virtual re-biomedicalisation, imposing the biomedical diagnostic and prognostic knowledge in a context where they are attempting to pursue alternative models of healing. This indicates a need to reassess conceptual arguments which engender an Internet-facilitated pluralism in medical knowledge, challenge to medical expertise or indeed process of patient empowerment (Goldstein, 2004; Hardey, 1999, 2002; Sharf, 1997).

Although further research is needed to confirm these observations, the Internet as a crucial pathway to CAM (e.g. Ernst and Schmidt, 2002; Schmidt and Ernst, 2004) also seems to be a largely erroneous proposition. Although there were patients in this study who used the Internet for such a purpose, the majority did not. Avoiding unnecessary exposure to biomedical diagnostic and prognostic information was often central to this process, thus problematising the potential role of the Internet as a source of biomedical *and* CAM-related information and support. A common theme was that, although it was possible to avoid biomedical knowledge on the Internet (i.e. selecting out specific sites rather than general searches), the temptation to type in 'Stage 2 breast cancer', for example, was often very strong despite the desire to transcend the sense of 'inevitability' (or indeed, depersonalisation) inherent in a biomedical prognosis (see Broom and Tovey, 2007a).

It seems that, in the light of these findings, attention is needed to the potential role of the Internet in establishing and reinforcing for individual patients the dominance and authority of biomedicine in UK cancer care. Although its potential for raising the profile of alternative therapeutics is certainly not lost, its potential for reinforcing biomedicine should be given equal attention. The desire of sociologists to promote a view of the liberation and empowerment of patients and non-biomedical stakeholders seems strong and this has been evident in Internet health studies hitherto. However, the role of the Internet in reinforcing the status quo, or indeed propagating biomedical conceptions of disease and the body, has received relatively little attention despite increasing recognition that early Internet studies over estimated its fundamentally reformative nature, and largely ignored differentiation in experience at a grassroots level (e.g. Broom, 2005; Henwood *et al.*, 2003).

It should be emphasised that, in making this argument, we do not mean to deny the usefulness of the Internet to many cancer patients or the usefulness of the early Internet studies that emphasised these positive features of new information technologies in healthcare. Rather, our intention is to break down some of the myths that have been built up around the Internet both within the sociological literature and in the biomedical literature and which ultimately misrepresent patient experience and the implications of the Internet for differently positioned stakeholders.

3 Integrating CAM

A comparative analysis of hospice versus hospital medicine

Introduction

The integration of CAM raises considerable dilemmas regarding effectiveness within a medico-culture espousing EBM (Coulter, 2004), a professional body, which views much of the evidence available to back up CAM modalities as fundamentally flawed. However, huge public support and recent political pressure has meant that healthcare providers cannot afford to ignore the needs of patients above and beyond biomedical cancer care. Responses to such demands have been varied and large sections of UK cancer services remain largely biomedical in approach. However, others are attempting some degree of (albeit limited) integration. As a result, individual organisations are facing a plenitude of dilemmas, including the reassessment of traditional notions of evidence and effectiveness.

This chapter moves to an examination of the specific *organisational* issues and responses that emerge in the context of the provision of CAM to cancer patients. In particular, we compare two quite different contexts for the treatment of cancer patients: the hospice and the hospital. We focus here on how integration is managed in each organisation, examining professional boundary disputes and inter-professional dynamics. Of particular interest are the rhetorical and practical strategies that are employed by a variety of differently positioned cancer clinicians (i.e. palliative care specialists and medical oncologists) to negotiate the complexities of the interface of CAM and biomedicine. Before discussion of the specific results of this inter-organisational comparison, some background on the nature of evidence in medicine and in oncology is useful to contextualise our analysis.

EBM and the evidence hierarchy

The EBM movement began to develop in the 1970s, and solidified as a key concept in health policy in the 1990s (Timmermans and Kolker, 2004). In the last decade, aided by the proliferation of EBM centres and international stakeholders (e.g. the Cochrane Collaboration), EBM has received increasing attention from health social scientists internationally as a crucial contemporary social movement (e.g. Barry, 2006; Goldenberg, 2006; Jackson and Scambler, 2007; Lambert, 2006; Mykhalovskiy and Weir, 2004; Villanueva-Russell, 2005; Willis and White, 2002). The EBM movement has resulted in other policy trajectories, including the development of EBP (Banning, 2005), and there have also been attempts in the US to establish EBCAM (evidence-based CAM) centres and research groups (e.g. Hardy *et al.*, 2001; Wilson and Mills, 2002). This process of applying the principles of EBM to CAM has been limited in success due to the lack of existing RCT-based studies of CAMs; lack of money and expertise to do such studies; and a continuing belief within the CAM community that paradigmatic issues fuel opposition to their practices, not the evidence base available.

Social scientists have regularly criticised EBM as, among other things, a threat to doctor/patient communication and the value and integrity of individual clinical judgement (Goldenberg, 2006; Mykhalovskiy, 2003; Pope, 2003). Moreover, EBM has been criticised for a failure to address grassroots processes within complex healthcare environments (Mendelson and Carino, 2005). Social theorists have also pointed out the naivety of positivist empiricism, particularly in terms of the lack of acknowledgement of the influence of values on knowledge and fact production (e.g. Goldenberg, 2006). Further weight is added to such arguments given the fact that there is no evidence that EBM actually improves outcomes for patients, and, furthermore, there is considerable doubt that teaching clinicians the principals of EBM, in its current form, actually benefits patients (Dobbie *et al.*, 2000; Morrison *et al.*, 1999).

Regardless of arguments about success or failure, the notion of EBM is omnipresent in UK healthcare policy and, indeed, in the accounts of the clinicians' interviewed here. A central tenet of EBM is the biomedical hierarchy of evidence, which is broadly as follows: (1) systematic reviews with meta-analysis; (2) experimental studies (e.g. randomised controlled trials);[1] (3) quasi-experimental studies (e.g. before-and-after studies); (4) observational studies (e.g. cohort study); (5) descriptive studies (e.g. case series); and (6) interpretivist studies (e.g. qualitative interview studies) (see Broom *et al.*, 2004). Moreover, certain study designs are considered, by clinical epidemiologists, only to be able to measure *accurately* certain facets of healthcare. An RCT is viewed as able to measure the effectiveness of an intervention; a case control/cohort measures harm; a cross-sectional study measures cause (aetiology) and prevalence; a cohort study measures prognosis; and a qualitative study, meaning.

This hierarchy of evidence has been employed rigorously by organisations like the Cochrane Collaboration and is viewed by the majority of the biomedical community as crucial for rating the quality of clinical evidence. It is, if you like, the epistemological schema which defines what constitutes good knowledge and effectiveness; a schema that is employed both rhetorically and practically at a grassroots level by many biomedical clinicians.

In practice, as illustrated by the data presented in the next section, treatment and funding decisions do not necessarily follow the ideals espoused by the biomedical community. At a grassroots level, decision-making is often more complicated and subjective (see also Passik and Kirsh, 2000; Tredaniel *et al.*, 2005), study designs often do not reach the gold standard, and informal systems operate in NHS Trusts that influence the treatment choices made available to patients.

EBM: research in the oncology setting

There is little research examining the degree to which oncology treatments are evidence based. The exception is a study by Foy *et al.* (1999) which examined the evidence threshold for oncology treatments provided by an NHS Trust in Manchester. This study found that treatment funding was influenced not just by the level of evidence available, but also by the value placed on certain clinical outcomes by particular individual consultants, political pressure and financial pressure. Moreover, Foy *et al.* (1999) discovered that the level of evidence was often below the biomedical gold standard (i.e. meta-analysis of multiple randomised controlled trials). This is not particularly surprising in itself, but what was interesting was that a significant proportion of treatments were not backed up by randomised controlled trials at all (see also Burgers *et al.*, 2004; Djulbegovic and Sullivan, 1997; Djulbegovic *et al.*, 1999; Vincent and Djulbegovic, 2005).

Most practising medical oncologists rely on systematic reviews for clinical decision-making (the supposed highest level of clinical evidence), but yet studies have shown the fundamental flaw in assumptions about the quality of available reviews. For example, a study by Vigna-Taglianti *et al.* (2006) examined 80 so-called 'reviews', 36 focusing on breast and 44 on colorectal cancer. Twenty-three reviews (29 per cent) did not match the definition of systematic review. In 17 (21 per cent) the searching methods were unclear or described elsewhere. Forty (50 per cent) were systematic. Not systematic, low- and very low-quality reviews accounted for 70 per cent of the total. No review obtained the A+ class score; only 5 (6 per cent) the A−; and 7 (9 per cent) the B+. The results of this assessment provide a sober picture of the quality of the sources used to build guidelines (see also Cox, 2000).

The implication of this potential variability or evidence gap is significant, in terms of both the quality of biomedical cancer care and the potential integration of CAM into UK cancer services. If indeed the evidence hierarchy does not match grassroots processes, and informal systems operate within individual Trusts, awareness is needed of how these systems will affect attempts to get funding for CAM therapies.

Evidence and CAM

As outlined in Chapter 1, the sidelining of CAM in cancer care has often been justified by to the paucity of high-level evidence available. But what is the actual evidence base for CAM, if any? A review of the literature illustrates considerable differentiation in the evidence base available for particular CAMs (Ernst, 2001a). RCTs have shown that acupuncture and acupressure are practical, safe and inexpensive ways of reducing nausea and vomiting after cancer treatment (e.g. Ernst, 2001; Filshie, 1990). Forms of spiritual healing (e.g. reiki and therapeutic touch) and mindfulness-based stress reduction have also been shown in clinical trials to lower anxiety, enhance quality of life and improve overall wellbeing in cancer patients (see Carlson *et al.*, 2004; Ernst, 2001a; Tavares, 2003). However, other CAM therapies provided in the institutions examined in this study, such as aromatherapy, massage and reflexology, have little high-level biomedical evidence to back up their efficacy in cancer care (Corner *et al.*, 1995; Soden *et al.*, 2004; Stephenson *et al.*, 2000).

Advocates argue that many CAMs involve highly complex interventions that rely heavily on psychosocial outcomes that cannot easily be assessed in a controlled trial. It has also been argued that outcomes are highly subjective and cannot easily be measured in biomedical study designs. Even the strongest proponents of applying the evidence hierarchy to CAM acknowledge that a double-blind design to compare, for example, aromatherapy treatments is probably impossible to achieve (e.g. Cooke and Ernst, 2000). However, they also argue that the CAM community needs to do much more in terms of producing high-quality evidence in order to play a more central role in the UK cancer services (see also Adams, 2007).

Evidence and organisational setting: the hospice and the hospital

As evidenced in the results of the current study shown below, processes of integration (or barriers limiting it) are not linear and internal procedures vary depending on the organisational context. Hospices in the UK have been at the forefront of offering holistic care to cancer patients (see Tavares, 2003). Research has indicated that within the hospice setting doctors tend to focus more on treatment of the whole person (i.e. subjective spiritual and emotional needs), in contrast to the disease focus evident in hospital oncology settings (Addington-Hall and Karlsen, 2005). Studies of nurses working in hospice settings also illustrate a focus on overall patient wellbeing and pursuing a holistic approach to palliation (e.g. Chiu and Mok, 2004). Given this specific context, it seems possible that biomedical constructions of evidence may play less of a role within the hospice than meeting patients' subjective needs at the end of life, particularly given the fact that evidence for palliative care interventions has historically been poor due to difficulties researching terminally ill patients (Bain *et al.*, 2003). Therapeutic modalities, traditionally marginalised in biomedical cancer care (e.g. reiki, reflexology and spiritual healing), may be assessed less in terms of physiological, observable effect and more according to subjective measures related to patient satisfaction with care and overall wellbeing.

However, as is illustrated by the results of the current study, it is not simply a matter of hospices and palliative care clinicians being more open to CAM and integrative medicine. Despite taking a very different approach from that of the hospital staff in terms of how they perceive the role of CAM, the hospice staff also have to negotiate a complex array of pressures when attempting to provide quality care to cancer patients, and, indeed, are also subject to biomedical parameters espousing evidence-based medicine.

The hospital

As distinct from the hospice setting, hospital-based oncology services have traditionally focused on cure rates and disease reduction, in part due to the terminal nature of many cancers and societal demand for curative treatments. Although oncology as a medical speciality has extended beyond the purely disease-centred approach to care seen in the mid-twentieth century (J. Turner *et al.*, 2005), there is still little direct integration of CAM with oncology services in the UK, and, significantly, neither general medical nor oncology specialist training involves significant education on CAM treatments (Murdoch-Eaton and Crombie, 2002). At present, there is very little direct NHS funding for CAM therapies for cancer patients. Currently funding comes almost exclusively from the volunteer sector or services are offered free of charge by individual CAM therapists.

In terms of integrating CAMs, the hospital setting is very different from that of the hospice, with a history of evidence and disease reduction as central to funding decision-making. Given the rhetoric of, and attempts at implementing, EBM and arguments regarding the lack of evidence to back up many CAMs (House of Lords, 2000), there exists considerable potential for conflict regarding integration within the hospital context (Coulter, 2004). A key focus of this study was examining how these two very different healthcare environments outlined above (and the clinicians working within them) are approaching the increased presence of CAM and the demand for it from cancer patients.

Organisational dynamics in theoretical context

For sociologists, the integration of CAM in cancer care (or lack thereof) raises considerable theoretical concerns. On the one hand, the increased presence of CAM presents a potential challenge to, and threatens reconfiguration of, established biomedical organisational culture. As integration becomes increasingly common, paradigmatically distinct practices will increasingly interact together and, effectively, compete for resources. Moreover, in the current context, in which biomedical cancer treatments still maintain a virtual monopoly, the integration of CAM potentially challenges (but is not necessarily changing) the biomedical culture of NHS cancer facilities, potentially contesting the philosophical ideals and assumptive base of biomedicine.

It could be argued that the introduction of CAMs for cancer patients offers a challenge to the symbolic power of the medical profession (Boon *et al.*, 2004), potentially reconstructing them as one of a number of cancer clinicians and, furthermore, potentially questioning the central tenets of their epistemological/ideological position. Moreover, the increased integration of CAM within the NHS could be seen as contributing, among other factors, to the deprofessionalisation of biomedicine (Haug, 1973, 1988). In this context, as outlined in the Introduction, the process of deprofessionalisation denotes a demystification of medical expertise and increasing lay scepticism about biomedical health professionals. This process of deprofessionalisation is seen to result from reductions in the monopolisation of esoteric knowledge, autonomy in work performance and authority over clients (Haug, 1973, 1988). But are such arguments relevant to what is happening at the point of delivery in cancer services?

The proliferation of CAM has to a certain degree catalysed a movement towards a market or consumerist model of healthcare, increasing the range of options available to consumers, encouraging patients to question biomedical advice and potentially challenging the monopoly of biomedicine in healthcare delivery (Bombardieri and Easthope, 2000). Furthermore, the increased consumption of CAM by patients has been seen as part of a broader movement towards a questioning of the benefits of the primacy of biomedicine in health provision and as a challenge to doctors' clinical authority (e.g. Lupton, 1997).

However, and as outlined in the Introduction, such a binary analysis is increasingly criticised by sociologists who recognise the complexity of grassroots organisational processes and the importance of intra-professional differentiation (e.g. Timmermans and Kolker, 2004). They warn against constructing an oversimplified view of the waxing or waning of the biomedical profession (e.g. Broom, 2005; Germov, 1995; Timmermans and Kolker, 2004). For example, Lewis *et al.* (2003) argue that the so-called loss of professional autonomy in medicine may be viewed more as an adjustment to the current social context rather than a breakdown in professional control. Similarly, as evidenced in the results presented below, the notion of CAM as a 'challenge' to biomedicine is inadequate to capture the complex strategies being used by both medics and CAM therapists to construct (and maintain) their own validity in particular organisational settings.

As such, we argue below that based on the results of our research a more nuanced approach is needed to examine how the integration of CAM is managed by different actors, what *specific* position CAMs are allowed to occupy within particular organisational settings and the mechanics of how such roles are negotiated or indeed enforced. In particular, insight is needed into clinicians' relationships with, and responses to, potential CAM integration to actually discover what is occurring at the point of service delivery. We know little about whether (and in what ways) CAMs and biomedicine are being shaped by processes of integration, and about the implications for professional identities and therapeutic processes. In order to engage with such issues, in this chapter we move past oversimplified binary constructions of the relationship between CAM and biomedicine to examine the mechanisms through which integration is managed, reflecting on the implications for CAM in cancer care, within and between different organisational contexts.

Description of the two organisational case studies

Hospital

The NHS teaching hospital that we examined has one of the largest cancer treatment facilities in the north of England. It has innovative facilities for providing support (both social and informational) and CAMs to cancer patients, through a centre set up and funded by the volunteer sector and located in the centre of the hospital site. These services are rationed, with most patients placed on a waiting list and limited to six courses of each CAM therapy (this is adjusted, with patients pushed up the waiting list depending on their stage of disease). The CAM therapists are volunteers, offering, generally, one day a week of their time to provide their therapy free to cancer patients. The coordinator (a qualified nurse) of the centre makes the decision, in collaboration with hospital management, about which therapists can operate in the centre. Patients technically have to 'get the OK' from their oncologist to receive a CAM therapy (see results on pp. 63–75 for discussion on this process) but the degree to which this is enforced remains ambiguous.

Hospice

The hospice we selected provides patients with an array of CAM therapies, including acupuncture, reiki, massage, hypnotherapy, reflexology and aromatherapy (although these change depending on the availability of practitioners and internal audits of patients' responses to the service). Furthermore, due to the volunteer status of most CAM practitioners (other than the coordinator), there is a relatively high turnover of staff. The majority of the patients at the hospice are cancer patients. The two palliative care consultants effectively supervise all treatments offered in the hospice, although a manager oversees the whole organisation. Although the hospice receives some NHS funding, there is a historical separation (albeit implicit rather than policy directed) between the hospice movement and the NHS, and, furthermore, the hospice receives almost half its funding from public donations. Thus, there is a degree of autonomy (at least from the primary care trust) in the hospice movement, resulting, as we see below, in quite different strategies to integrate CAM.

The hospital context: evidence, effectiveness and the biomedical gold standard

Questions about what constitutes evidence and clinical effectiveness have been at the core of debates about CAM and biomedicine. In particular, debate has centred on several key issues such as how effectiveness should (or can) be measured; the degree to which biomedicine actually practises EBM; and the reasons why a biomedical-type evidence base does not exist to back up many CAM practices. Within this study we were interested in exploring who determines what constitutes good evidence at a grassroots level; how far up the evidence hierarchy evidence has to be in oncology before a treatment is actually funded; and whether informal systems exist that shape decision-making.

In order to explore such issues, the clinicians were asked to talk about what they viewed as constituting validity and effectiveness, in their words, and in their specific organisational context. As seen in the excerpts presented below, the process of a treatment being considered by the management, getting funded and being viewed as effective in an NHS Trust is a much more subjective and complex process than the judgement of whether an intervention merely is evidence based:

INTERVIEWER: How do you personally assess the validity of a treatment?

MEDICAL ONCOLOGIST: We have this sort of grading system for our evidence base which you are probably aware of, and we use this more and more now, where the best evidence is the meta-analysis or . . . systematic review and meta-analysis where available, randomised control trials and so on . . . That's the sort of relationship of trust within the Trust, that we won't use unproven therapies.

INTERVIEWER: What does unproven mean? Have all your treatments had Phase 3 clinical trials, or even randomised controlled trials?

MEDICAL ONCOLOGIST: Absolutely not and that's a good point. A lot of things that we do that are not supported by the highest grade of evidence and that may be because we have been unable to gather that evidence. It may be because they are very rare conditions in which case you use the next best . . .

INTERVIEWER: So ultimately, would hospital policy exclude all complementary therapies . . . because there is no evidence?

MEDICAL ONCOLOGIST: You do not have to have a meta-analysis or even a randomised controlled trial, but you would have to present available evidence and convince the hospital management . . . It would depend on why the evidence is not there; how likely is this treatment to be toxic; how expensive it is likely to be . . . even who [which specialist] is asking for the treatment to be funded and their reputation.

(male, 43 years, research and clinical)

A specialist cancer nurse:

SPECIALIST BREAST CANCER NURSE: Hospitals are still very much medical model orientated, so you only start doing something new when there is good evidence for it . . . Now at some point somebody says, 'We have got this pot of money, how are we going to spend it? Are we going to bring in this new drug that we know cures so many people because someone has done some trials or are we going to pay for some foot massage?' It depends how clever that person is who presents the argument.

(female, 46 years, clinical specialist nurse)

The above excerpts illustrate the highly complex and subjective process of achieving funding and legitimacy within an NHS cancer facility. Like the majority of the other specialists interviewed, the specialist shown above begins with an ideal; an ideal that diminishes in relevance in practice. Getting funded, as he acknowledges, is influenced by professional status, the availability of funds and how convincing an individual specialist is; not merely the level of evidence presented to the Trust. What emerged from the specialists' accounts was considerable disparity between the ideal of evidence-based medicine and actual organisational practices. Regardless of this discrepancy between policy and practice, idealised notions of the biomedical evidence base were still central to the delineation of CAM and biomedicine. As will be seen later in this discussion, such idealised constructions of biomedicine also provide a discursive basis for justifying organisational processes delimiting the provision (or delivery) of CAM.

The biomedical hierarchy of evidence exists to ensure that a high standard is met *if possible*, and clearly some flexibility must exist to ensure patient care is not compromised, particularly in cases of rare conditions where experimental studies are impossible (let alone RCTs). However, this ideal is not applied across the board but, rather, in some instances, it is used to deny treatments funding and legitimacy in cases where clinicians are not well placed to negotiate this rather subjective and political process (i.e. CAM therapists).

The system, as outlined by a number of the specialists interviewed here, can be flexible if the desire to be flexible exists, but there is a default position if management does not view treatments as appropriate. This position is that in cases where any doubt exists regarding the logic behind the treatment (i.e. its paradigmatic base) it must reach the so-called gold standard. This may pose significant difficulties when treatments are perceived to be paradigmatically incommensurable with the biomedical model, a model which clearly underpins the informal system outlined above.

This 'black box' of funding decision-making has considerable implications for the integration of CAM into NHS hospitals. Hitherto, the biomedical community has maintained that CAM cannot be integrated unless a high level of evidence is presented (e.g. Ernst, 2000). However, the subjective process of decision-making regarding many biomedical cancer treatments suggests that CAM therapies may also have to achieve more than a high level of scientific evidence to receive funding and clinical legitimacy. Questions like is the clinician a scientist, does she/he have a scientific mind and is there bio-medically justifiable logic behind the treatment may be just as important as clinical evidence.

The importance of the scientific mind

Despite the biomedical ideal of evidence-based medicine, and the tendency of these specialists to utilise this rhetorically in their accounts of CAM, there was also an acknowledgement that a large proportion of biomedical cancer treatments that get funded do not actually meet their organisation's own criteria for establishing effectiveness. Effectiveness, according to these special-ists, would often be established retrospectively. For example, the trial would begin after the intervention was funded by the Trust and the intervention would be dropped or use would continue depending on the outcome of the study. What was particularly interesting was the way in which 'a scientific mind' was viewed by all the hospital-based medical specialists as a reasonable sub-stitute for a lack of high-grade evidence. As suggested above, such factors are pragmatic in the sense that they are focused on allowing biomedical treat-ments (with limited evidence available) into the system, rather than slippage across the board (i.e. allowing all therapies through, including CAMs):

MEDICAL ONCOLOGIST: I wouldn't support the use of public money to use therapies that are not evidence based. Not being, you know, any attempt at really providing an evidence base, and some of the stuff that we do here hasn't got a very good evidence base, but it's at least within an environment which is sceptical of its own treatments and, you know, looking to make an evidence base if it can and quite happy to disregard treatments that are of no benefit. That kind of scepticism is maybe the important aspect of modern medicine which is perhaps not an aspect of complementary medicine. I think it would be difficult to argue for the use of public money for complementary medicines personally.

(male, 43 years, research and clinical)

As can be seen from this excerpt, the scientific mind and scepticism are used rhetorically to delineate between CAM therapists and doctors, and to justify treatment decision-making. Again, there is an acknowledgement of a lack of evidence for many biomedical cancer treatments. However, the poten-tial blurring of boundaries resulting from the realisation that biomedicine is not as evidenced based as it claims to be is countered by a delineation of CAM and biomedical clinicians through constructions of what constitutes a rational, scientific mind.

We were also interested in the biomedical clinicians' views on how they would react if scientific evidence was available for complementary therapies. It emerged that although they claimed they would accept this knowledge if it was scientifically legitimate (i.e. published in the right journals, with an appropriate methodological design, vetted by the right people and so on), they viewed this as an implausible scenario:

INTERVIEWER: What if we could show you good evidence on the effectiveness of a complementary therapy?
MEDICAL ONCOLOGIST: Well, I suppose we'd use it, but . . . for most complementary things there is never going to be the evidence. If they actually worked, I think we would probably already know about it . . . occasionally things slip through like acupuncture but this is an exception.

(female, 43 years, research and clinical)

Another respondent:

MEDICAL ONCOLOGIST: [Complementary therapies] are inspirational therapies . . . you know, somebody has an idea about something that would work and it hasn't been through a process of scientific validation . . . they [aren't] therapeutic, like more supportive. They certainly aren't coming from the deep world-view that we have developed through scientific experimentation . . . and realistically there's unlikely to be any evidence produced for it either.

(male, 43 years, medical oncologist)

Although there was acknowledgement that treatments would have to be considered if evidence was available (and that some CAM treatments like acupuncture had actually been scientifically proven), there was considerable scepticism in terms of whether there would ever be enough evidence for most modalities even to warrant serious consideration.

In part, this may be linked to the views of many CAM therapists about what evidence is actually necessary to achieve validity. In this study the CAM therapists largely rejected the necessity of high-level evidence, prioritising intuition and anecdote:

INTERVIEWER: How do you assess whether a treatment or a therapy is effective? How important is scientific evidence?
CAM THERAPIST: Not very. I assess effectiveness by the physical responses of the clients and also the sort of feedback that they will give you at the end of the sessions and the fact that they want to come back for more.

(female, 58 years, aromatherapy/massage)

Another respondent:

INTERVIEWER: For you, what do you feel is evidence?
CAM THERAPIST: Patient comfort, I think, and wellbeing. It's very difficult to put your finger on . . . Well, we've got written evidence because we keep records and there's the patients or clients that you see. That's visible . . . that's evidence to me.

(female, age not stated, aromatherapy/massage)

Thus we see quite different views of what constitutes evidence from the perspective of the CAM therapists. In terms of the hierarchy of evidence outlined previously, the medical oncologists are operating (at least rhetorically) from the top of the ladder (meta-analysis), whereas the CAM therapies espouse a subjective, individualised view of effectiveness (more aligned to the interpretivist traditions in research design). Thus, ontologically and epistemologically they are operating at very different ends of the spectrum; a schism that, as suggested by the oncologists above, makes it less likely that CAM modalities will produce the kind of evidence necessary to warrant consideration for direct funding by the NHS.

However, the objectives of the CAM therapists also differed from those of the oncologists, with a focus on aspects of cancer care like patient comfort, lowering stress and anxiety, and reducing pain and nausea. As one CAM therapist suggested, 'as long as we are doing no harm, I don't think evidence really matters'. However, for the oncologists it was not the objective of the CAM treatment that was crucial, but rather the scientific logic behind the intervention. Compromising on the level of evidence, based on the specific claims being made about the treatment (e.g. supportive or calming rather than curative), was viewed as a form of slippage away from the ideal of evidence-based practice.

Given the arguments presented thus far, we were interested in these oncologists' views on the provision of CAM to patients in their hospital and how they interacted (if at all) with the support centre and the CAM therapists operating within it. Of specific interest, given the rhetoric of evidence-based practice, were their views on the fact that their hospital was providing therapies that were not supported by biomedically defined scientific evidence.

Getting CAM in the back door

A key argument amongst the medical community, justifying the delimiting of many CAM modalities, has been the ethical practice of only treating patients when high-quality evidence is available, although we have already seen the rather subjective nature of this concept of being evidence based. Our concern in this study was not so much this double standard in relation to the need for evidence. Rather, it was how the clinical staff made sense of the fact that their Trust offers cancer patients a range of CAM therapies despite this ethical practice. As we see in the next excerpt, the clinical staff (and the hospital management) had developed a series of rationalisations which allowed them to avoid addressing what might be a clear deviation from the rhetoric (and organisational policy) of evidence-based medicine and, perhaps more importantly, from subjecting CAMs to the same processes of legitimation as biomedical treatments (thereby potentially denying a highly popular service to cancer patients):

INTERVIEWER: Out of interest, how did the [complementary] therapies in the

[name of hospital centre] get passed by the hospital management if
they . . .
MEDICAL ONCOLOGIST: Well, they are not being paid for by . . .
INTERVIEWER: So they have no ethical responsibility?
MEDICAL ONCOLOGIST: That's a very good question. Yes, they are not seen
as therapies offered by the hospital.
INTERVIEWER: They are offered to every cancer patient that goes in there?
MEDICAL ONCOLOGIST: Yes, but not by the Trust. The [volunteer-sector
organisation] is providing an environment and often those therapists are
offering that service for free.
INTERVIEWER: So the hospital has no ethical obligations if it has not been
paid for?
MEDICAL ONCOLOGIST: Correct. If it is not being seen to be delivered by
the Trust.

(male, 43 years, research and clinical)

In this excerpt we see the way in which this particular Trust, and its oncologists, pragmatically draw a line between what it provides and what it does not
provide to patients. This strategy of demarcation (i.e. Trust sanctioned/not
Trust sanctioned) has both a potentially positive and negative impact for
CAM therapies and therapists. On the one hand, it allows CAM therapists
to operate in the hospital system (at least geographically) and get a foothold
in cancer care within the hospital premises. However, it also isolates them,
financially and professionally, giving them a right to treat, but not the right
to legitimacy within the hospital system. Thus we see a kind of pseudo-
integration whereby CAMs are allowed in the back door. This idea of turning
a blind eye also emerged in the interviews with the nurses:

SPECIALIST BREAST CANCER NURSE: My response is invariably going to be
if that is something that you want to do, then go for it. They are not
going to let them have anything at the [centre] that the consultant isn't
going to be happy with . . . and if they do, then I don't want to know
about it. [laughs]

(female, 46 years, clinical specialist nurse)

As well as organisational strategies to accommodate (but not encourage)
integration the medical specialists interviewed also utilised particular strategies to limit the clinical legitimacy of the CAM therapists working in the
hospital. As evidenced in the excerpts below, and in the interviews with the
clinicians, there was a deliberate policy of unspoken disapproval combined
with a strategy of accommodation in the medical consultation. Moreover,
particular strategies were employed to prevent communication between the
CAM therapists and the consultants, which ultimately formed one part of a
deliberate process of professional distancing:

MEDICAL ONCOLOGIST: I don't refer people for any, like, complementary therapies but I point people sometimes in the direction of the [hospital-based CAM centre] for the support of things it has on offer and mention that there are things available there.

INTERVIEWER: What's the difference between 'referral' and 'mention'?

MEDICAL ONCOLOGIST: I suppose it would be about me . . . I think a 'referral' is if I actually wrote to a practitioner with details about a patient and said, 'Please see this patient with whom I've discussed X, Y, Z.'

(female, 48 years, research and clinical)

Another respondent:

MEDICAL ONCOLOGIST: I wouldn't refer anyone there. I wouldn't stop them but I wouldn't refer them either.

(male, 43 years, research and clinical)

Another respondent:

CAM THERAPIST: We write to every consultant of every new referral and we very rarely get a response, you know, saying that this person has been either self-referred or has been referred, and just if they have any issues, will they let us know, but we hardly ever get a response . . . they don't acknowledge us here.

(female, 58 years, aromatherapist)

None of the oncologists interviewed said they would be willing to refer a patient for CAM as this would signify a formal network between them and the CAM therapists, but also it would signify support for the clinical legitimacy of the CAM practices offered. The majority would not mention the hospital's support (and CAM) centre to patients, but some would be willing to discuss it if the patient brought it up. Moreover, as one specialist said, 'If I suggest they go there, then clearly I'm saying these things are effective. Well, I can't say that.' Ethics, in this context, albeit implicitly, is used to rationalise professional distancing.

As is illustrated by the results presented thus far, there are considerable barriers to the provision of CAM to patients in the hospital setting, with organisational and individual strategies to limit integration and the legitimacy of CAM practices. Ethics, evidence and the scientific mind are used both to delineate discursively and to delimit practically the integration of CAM in the hospital setting. Although on the surface there is apparent integration (i.e. existence of a CAM centre), there is little or no involvement between the biomedical services and the CAM services within this hospital. Moreover, internal procedures and individual practitioners are actively limiting the integration of CAM therapies into UK cancer services. It is clearly the case that acceptance of treatments and treatment funding decisions, in this context, is not merely about having the evidence available, as per the biomedical ideal. Rather, the paradigmatic underpinnings of a particular modality are vital and informal systems develop within organisations to delimit practices that are incommensurable with the biomedical paradigm.

The hospice context: balancing public support, clinical legitimacy and religiosity

Whilst the hospital staff were concerned about levels of evidence and clinical efficacy, the hospice staff took a very different approach to integration. Rather than focusing on the biomedical hierarchy of evidence, concerns amongst the hospice staff and management were orientated around providing a comfortable, holistic environment for patients and meeting public needs. However, maintaining public donations was also an important factor driving decision-making and there was considerably more pressure to provide a range of therapeutic modalities to be competitive with other hospices. CAM therapies were seen to bolster the legitimacy of the hospice's approach to end-of-life care, regardless of the level of evidence available to justify their provision. However, within this organisational context there was considerable concern regarding the ideological basis of certain CAM modalities and the potential of CAM therapies to disrupt prevailing belief systems such as Christianity:

PALLIATIVE CARE SPECIALIST: We have got to toe a very sort of very middle path with [complementary therapies] because, you know, we have to both be encouraging with new therapies . . . but at the same time, we have to also, you know, protect our reputation so to speak.
INTERVIEWER: Is it tied to funding?
PALLIATIVE CARE SPECIALIST: Yes, you know the PCT [Primary Care Trust] might have a comment on [CAM] but unlikely. It is more likely to be that the public are saying, 'Well, how come you are providing this?' and that may impact on public donations to the hospice, which we rely on. Also there is religious element, remember; this hospice was founded by [religious organisation], so there is quite, you know, some people who are extreme in their religious views – they almost see this, you know, complementary therapy, as being, you know . . .
INTERVIEWER: Evil?
PALLIATIVE CARE SPECIALIST: Akin to the devil, it's the devil itself, so, you know, we have to also be mindful of those sorts of things.
(male, 39 years, hospice management)

Hospices have to negotiate very different issues in relation to the integration of CAM. Securing funding drives decision-making significantly more than in the hospital setting and, furthermore, the resistance of the PCT (Primary Care Trust) to intervening in palliative care services means that there is limited political pressure put on the hospice to either integrate or limit the integration of CAM. Moreover, a degree of separation from the bureaucratic structures of the NHS means that the biomedical evidence hierarchy can be more easily sidelined as a driving force behind funding decision-making, and can be replaced by a more patient-centred focus on individualised, subjective outcomes.

It was evident that popularist demand for different modalities drove hospice decision-making much more than the hospital setting. Moreover, religious roots (particularly given the Christian roots of the hospice movement) and community beliefs create a very different set of pressures from those experienced by the hospital staff. Death has traditionally been associated with religiosity, and given the fact that a large proportion of UK citizens consider themselves religious (ONS, 2001), great sensitivity is needed, by the hospice, to ensure that prevailing religious values are upheld, whilst providing a holistic approach to end-of-life care. CAMs have long been at odds with the more fundamentalist Christian belief systems (Melton, 2001), particularly evangelical Pentecostalism, and thus offering CAMs espousing new age or alternative transcendental values potentially creates problems for the hospice.

In large part, as illustrated later in this discussion (pp. 73–4), this particular hospice manages these potential paradigm clashes (regarding both religious values and the biomedical model) through tight controls on discussion about the ideological facets of the CAMs delivered and the ways in which CAM therapists are allowed to interact with, and represent their therapies to, patients. This has important implications in terms of the potential translation (see Star and Griesemer, 1989) of CAMs within the hospice, such as the weakening of ideological bases and the biomedicalisation of CAM practitioners. As discussed below, the enlistment of selected CAMs within the hospice movement may have unintended implications for CAM modalities as biomedics select particular practices and types of individuals to deliver them, and in the process influence the very character of the therapeutic process.

The nature of palliative care

Another important influence on the nature of CAM integration in the hospice relates to the nature of palliative care. Many existing biomedical palliative care treatments are not evidence-based due to the immense difficulties involved in constructing clinical trials of patients near death (Bain *et al.*, 2003). The biomedical hierarchy of evidence, espoused by the hospital-based oncologists interviewed, is simply impractical within this context, resulting in a institutionally specific reassessment of what constitutes a *high enough* level of evidence. For example, as stated by the palliative care specialists interviewed here, there is considerable experimentation with new regimens if standard treatments are not effective in relieving pain – a flexibility not seen to this degree in the hospital system. In this context, anecdotal evidence, clinical judgement and adaptation to the patient are central to palliative care (Bain *et al.*, 2003). Few palliative care interventions have been subject to randomised controlled trials, let alone systematic reviews, and palliative care clinical practice has something of an affinity with particular forms of evidence which in the biomedical hierarchy are low. This places palliative care much closer to CAM in the hierarchy of evidence (i.e. largely backed up by observational studies) and in its ontological and epistemological positioning, with considerable implications for how CAM is viewed in this context:

PALLIATIVE CARE SPECIALIST: We work in the field of palliative medicine, where we use a lot of drugs that are not licensed, but we use them, and the evidence on which we use them is little and small. I have got loads of examples where we use drugs where there has been two case reports that have been published, but we have used it because we are struggling to find a solution, and the cost, the burden, seems low and the potential benefits seem considerable, then do it. It's the same process I think with complementary therapies because you know the evidence isn't going to be there.

INTERVIEWER: So what about ethical practice, as a clinician, to treat the patients with the best or most effective treatment and minimise any risk?

PALLIATIVE CARE SPECIALIST: ... the patient is at the heart of the decision-making and therefore there may be interventions or manoeuvres that we do which can't be justified by evidence, but which, when put in the context of that individual patient, would seem wholly right, and that is exactly the same as complementary therapies.

INTERVIEWER: Some people would say that low-grade evidence is worse than no evidence at all; how would you respond to that?

PALLIATIVE CARE SPECIALIST: Some people would say high-grade evidence is worse than what you see in front of you.

(male, 39 years, hospice management)

This quotation, and many others during the interviews with the hospice clinicians, illustrates the very specific context of palliative care, and in particular how experiential knowledge and minimising harm become crucial aspects of decisions to offer particular treatments. The individual patients and how they respond to treatment come to the fore, and the rhetoric of EBM or EBP does not feature in their accounts. Thus, within this context, CAM is enlisted as another facet of a patient-centred approach to dying and palliation; a context in which evidence seems secondary to individual anecdote and clinician intuition.

We argue here that the concepts of *enlistment* and *translation* (central tenets of Actor-network theory) are useful for understanding the complex relationships between CAM, palliative medicine and hospital-based oncology. Actor-network theorists have consistently argued for a view of social order as given by the processes of establishing systems of difference, classification and category building, pursuing a relational way of understanding the world (see, for example, Latour, 1987, 1988, 1993, 1999, 1999a; Latour and Woolgar, 1979; Law, 1992, 1994, 1999). Their work has focused on the role of the human and the non-human (e.g. devices, texts or objects) in the activity of sorting, constituting the subject and cementing particular translations of events, entities and actions. Actor-network theorists have focused on local processes of ordering and resistance – relational processes of translation by which social order is constructed and reconstructed, or, put in another way, how durability within a given network is secured (Law, 1992) (e.g. humans, devices, texts or objects).

At an organisational level, this strategy of *enlisting* selected CAMs pragmatically secures the future of the hospice by being competitive and maintaining public funding. Integration thus forms one part of an organisational strategy to achieve relative durability and to secure its position within a network (Law, 1994). Moreover, there may be interplay between CAM integration and a desire for intra-professional differentiation in a historical context in which palliative care has been something of the black sheep amongst the medical specialties. Palliative specialists' enlistment of CAM, within their organisational context, may function as a means of intra-professional distinction, contributing to the legitimacy of palliative care by constructing it as a more patient-centred, open-minded and holistic sub-specialty of medicine. This process mirrors that seen in the nursing profession, with particular elements separating themselves out and using CAM as a method of intra-professional distinction and legitimation (Tovey and Adams, 2003).

Enlistment and translation of CAM in palliative care

However, as Star and Griesemer argue (1989), such processes of enlistment may have multiple and complex effects not necessarily intended by the original action. We argue similarly that, in the context of integration, the process of enlistment may actually inscribe CAM practices, potentially weakening their ideological base and delimiting the therapists' role in patient care. To illustrate this potential, within this hospice there were strict rules about how CAM therapists could relate to patients and, in particular, what role CAM therapists could play in patient care. CAM therapists were given clear instructions about the claims that could be made about the therapies they were providing, appropriate ways of describing them and what other aspects of care they could discuss:

INTERVIEWER: How do you decide what therapies to introduce?
COMPLEMENTARY THERAPY COORDINATOR/NURSE: We use the touch therapies . . . they are not an alternative health system so it is very much complementary . . . I am not a purist, we don't use the word healing, because then, if we use the word healing, we need to explain what we mean by healing regards about cure . . . I don't think there is a need to [go into] all the intricacies of the differences between reiki or spiritual healing or therapeutic touch. It is basically about explaining to patients what will happen head to toe . . . I am currently drawing up a patient information leaflet on reflexology. I initially talked about flushing the toxins out, but we had to take that out because that is just not our medicine here. For complementary therapies to advance in NHS-type settings we have to

take into account conventional healthcare professionals who might be reasonably sceptical about the claims complementary therapists make.

(female, age unknown, nurse)

Another CAM practitioner:

AROMATHERAPIST/MASSEUR: I think it is slightly different working at the hospice actually.

INTERVIEWER: How is it different?

AROMATHERAPIST/MASSEUR: Well, we actually sort of try to sort of help the patients come to terms with their illness really here and to try, in a way, to get them to talk a little bit . . . but, of course we don't give them any advice or anything like that.

INTERVIEWER: Why not give them any advice?

AROMATHERAPIST/MASSEUR: Well, we are not meant to really.

INTERVIEWER: No?

AROMATHERAPIST/MASSEUR: It's not part of our role to give advice.

INTERVIEWER: Is that what you have been told?

AROMATHERAPIST/MASSEUR: Yes.

INTERVIEWER: What constitutes advice?

AROMATHERAPIST/MASSEUR: Telling them treatments they should have or not have.

INTERVIEWER: Who tells you this?

AROMATHERAPIST/MASSEUR: [name of the coordinator].

(female, 59 years)

The complementary coordinator quoted above, who is also a nurse, instructed the CAM therapists, in consultation with the medical specialists, on their role and how they should relate to patients. This involved making sure that certain claims were not made to patients (i.e. ability to heal) and certain discussions were not had (i.e. what biomedical treatments they are on, and potential implications). In this way, clear boundaries are constructed between biomedical versus CAM clinicians' roles within the hospice. Moreover, in the job-interview process CAM therapists are quizzed on their skills, but also on what they believe their therapies can achieve. In this way, the medical staff carefully monitor both the CAM modality and its representation. Moreover, modalities viewed as explicitly counter to biomedical knowledge of the body were rejected, with the healing and touch therapies (which were represented as soothing and calming) preferred over more interventionist and diagnostic therapies (e.g. diets, supplements, herbalism, naturopathy, homeopathy).

As seen in the excerpts presented above, the organisational context of the hospice environment is distinct from that of the hospital, both in terms of the perspectives of the staff on what constitutes evidence and in terms of the ways in which CAM integration impacts on the success of the organisation as a whole. The evidence hierarchy is much less significant than patient and carer anecdotes about the success of the CAM therapies and the degree to which therapies are supported by the general public (feeding into donations). Organisationally, CAM therapies make the hospice stronger, and professionally the use of CAMs is not particularly ideologically threatening given the flexible and holistic approach espoused by the palliative care clinicians.

Discussion

In this chapter we have attempted to shed light on the complex processes involved in the integration of CAM in two organisational contexts. Our focus here has been on practitioners. This is of course not to deny the importance of other aspects of the integration process (e.g. the way in which patients act as drivers of change). They are simply beyond the scope of our discussions here.

The ways in which a range of differently positioned practitioners conceptualise and utilise evidence have been a key focus of this chapter. As such, the biomedical hierarchy of evidence provides a central conceptual framework for understanding dynamics at the point of CAM integration. This analytical schema sits at the core of the debates seen here regarding clinical effectiveness and professional legitimacy. As we have seen, the hierarchy of evidence – and its ontological and epistemological bases – forms the rationalisation for both clinical legitimacy and professional exclusion. However, the ways in which organisations (and medical specialties) view and utilise this hierarchy of evidence is not linear. In fact, how biomedical clinicians view evidence is variable and the ways in which CAM integration is occurring is organisationally specific. In this study it emerged that the structural characteristics of specific medical specialties mean that they have a greater or lesser affinity with different types of evidence (i.e. palliative care versus oncology), necessarily affecting their relationship with CAM.

In the hospital context examined here, biomedical clinicians employed discursive and regulatory strategies to delimit CAM integration and to delineate biomedicine and CAM treatments. Discourses of the evidence hierarchy, the superiority of scientific mind and being ethical formed a crucial part of professional gate-keeping. These clinicians' descriptions of their own profession (e.g. evidenced based, scientific, sceptical) and those of CAM (e.g. unscientific, inspirational, nice but unnecessary) represent a process of discursive delineation of CAM and biomedicine, justifying institutional fragmentation of CAM and biomedical treatments, and reinforcing the historical occupational control held by oncology consultants.

Such strategies of distinction on the part of these medical specialists have an element of justification in the sense that, regardless of the limitations of the evidence in oncology, higher levels of evidence do exist for biomedical cancer treatments. However, as seen in this study, this schism is exaggerated rhetorically (as a form of boundary work), but also it is often deployed uncritically with no sense of the ontological and epistemological tensions critical to understanding how knowledge and evidence are produced.

As well as methods of discursive delineation, organisational structures and informational practices have developed, at least within the Trust examined here, to ensure that CAMs can be provided but not legitimated, with rigid (albeit in policy only) frameworks and informal networks existing for introducing new treatments, preventing CAMs from gaining internal funding. Avoiding directing patients to CAM services and refusing to establish cross-referrals is a powerful way in which the oncologists restrict the role of CAM within the hospital setting.

In addition, by funding CAMs and delivering them through 'the back door', the volunteer sector effectively compensates for the refusal of clinical staff and the hospital management to address complex issues of effectiveness and the evidence-gap contradiction evident in their funding of some biomedical cancer treatments. Allowing CAM treatments to be delivered (or passive acceptance) is a pragmatic act by the Trust and probably improves patient care, but it also potentially undermines the legitimacy of the CAMs offered and the therapists involved. It also allows hospital management and staff to avoid dialogue about complex paradigmatic issues and methods of gauging effectiveness which could lead to increased continuity of care and more effective communication between CAM therapists and the biomedical clinicians.

The hospice staff, however, were distinctly *more* orientated towards patients' subjective needs, community support and inter-organisational competition. Rather than attempting to limit the integration of CAM as seen in the hospital setting, their strategy was to enlist (see Star and Griesemer, 1989) selected CAMs to boost the legitimacy of the hospice as a competitive environment for end-of-life care; a process made significantly easier by the low level of evidence available for their existing biomedical palliative treatments and the non-interventionist policy of the PCT.

However, in saying this, our data also showed that CAMs were closely regulated within the hospice, with only the healing and touch therapies provided due to perceptions of their benign and uncontroversial nature. Practices like homoeopathy and naturopathy were not offered due to their objectives (i.e. to actually treat disease rather than merely to alleviate pain or anxiety) and the need physically to consume treatments, illustrating considerable differentiation in how individual CAMs (with differing objectives and levels of evidence) are treated within this context. Tight control was maintained over claims-making by CAM practitioners, and nurses were placed in coordinating roles to restrict ideological claims and monitor the patient/ therapist relationship.

Star and Griesemer write about this process of strategic enlistment, arguing that entrepreneurs gradually enlist participants 'from a range of locations, re-interpret their concerns to fit their own pragmatic goal and then establish themselves as gatekeepers' (Star and Griesemer, 1989: 389). This process, they argue, occurs as actors negotiate with others within a given network, establishing alignments to build support and reinforce their position – a process that inevitably transforms both the enlister and the enlisted. Likewise, the integration of CAM in the hospice movement will ultimately influence the character, albeit in a limited way, of both CAM and palliative care medicine. Although integration may provide more exposure for certain CAM practices and practitioners, this process may fundamentally alter what is CAM and what it is to be a CAM practitioner (as well as the character of palliative care as a medical specialty), as particular actors seek to influence the character and representation of CAM practices, enlist certain modalities for their own goals and, in doing so, change the very nature of therapeutic practices.

For some of the CAM practitioners, operating within a biomedical context was something of a trade-off, in that, on the one hand, they gained a degree of professional legitimacy (a form of distinction from other CAM practitioners) but, on the other, they also lost a degree of professional autonomy and ideology. However, they also viewed their involvement as an opportunity to influence the nature of cancer and palliative care in the UK, inscribing their own perspectives of illness, death and wellbeing on the UK cancer services, as well as opening themselves to other actors' strategies of inscription and translation.

Conclusion

Given the results presented above, we argue that the integration of CAM should not be conceptualised as a mere challenge to biomedicine or as potentially contributing to this rather linear process of deprofessionalisation (a waning of biomedical authority). Rather, it should be seen as producing a complex array of responses, including evolving processes of strategic adaptation on the part of specialists and NHS organisations; processes that are organisationally specific and that do not necessarily represent a breakdown in biomedical clinicians' authority or status. Within the hospice, integration is actually key to the overall organisational goals and professional needs (i.e. offering competitive, holistic, populist care). As a result, biomedical clinicians working in this context, who perceive CAM as an inevitable (but not necessarily appropriate) part of cancer care, are finding ways to enlist (or shape) CAMs to complement their professional role and the strength of their organisation. Others, such as the clinicians in the hospital interviewed here, may view CAMs as a threat to their professional practices and biomedical ideological view, resulting in the deployment of particular discursive and regulatory strategies to delimit the integration, and expansion, of CAM services.

4 Oncologists' and specialist cancer nurses' approaches to CAM and their impact on patient action

Introduction

The inter-professional dynamics between CAM and biomedicine have been regularly examined within the sociological literature (e.g. Hirschkorn and Bourgeault, 2005; Mizrachi *et al.*, 2005). Such analyses have focused on the management of professional boundaries and the centrality of notions of evidence, efficacy and professionalism in shaping inter-professional dynamics. However, little is known about how inter- and intra-professional dynamics manifest at a grassroots level in clinical contexts and, importantly, how patients make sense of these and how they may impact on patient action. This paucity of research is particularly evident in cancer care, where ironically CAM use is the most prolific (e.g. Ernst and Cassileth, 1998; Lewith *et al.*, 2002; Rees *et al.*, 2000). In this specific disease context the responses of biomedical clinicians to patients' treatment preferences are of particular importance given the level of emotion and anxiety reported in treatment decision-making processes (see Arora, 2003; Hack *et al.*, 2005). Moreover, effective communication about CAM has been reported by both cancer patients and clinicians to enhance the patient/practitioner relationship (Roberts *et al.*, 2005).

Such patient–practitioner exchanges do not exist in a vacuum. Indeed, drawing on work from other areas of health research, the actual extent to which biomedical clinicians are actually pivotal to contemporary patient action on CAM is open to question. A plurality of information sources, such as the Internet (Broom, 2005), the influence of friends and family (Maly *et al.*, 2006) and the 'plurality of experts' (Giddens, 1990, 1991), evident in the CAM field are all characteristic of a multidimensional decision-making environment. In this context the impact and influence of those at the apex of formal legitimate authority (cancer specialists and, to a different extent, cancer nurses) require fresh empirical examination. Specifically, the chapter considers: (1) patient experience with cancer specialists and specialist cancer nurses about non-biomedical treatment options at this time of potential or actual 'integration'; (2) the impact of the attitudes and approach of biomedical practitioners on patient engagement with CAM; and (3) how processes are played out between oncologists and specialist nurses and how this impacts on patients.

The lay–professional interface in empirical and theoretical context

As outlined in the Introduction, the inter-professional dynamics between CAM and biomedicine have received significant attention from health sociologists over the last two decades. Key concerns have been the occupational dominance of biomedicine and the ongoing peripheralisation of many CAM modalities in the context of primary care (see Hirschkorn and Bourgeault, 2005). To a certain degree we have seen a gradual encroachment by CAM modalities such as acupuncture, chiropractic and osteopathy on biomedical territory for specific conditions (Kelner *et al.*, 2004). This has tended to occur in the context of chronic illness and pain-related conditions requiring manipulation. Most CAM practitioners are still reliant on private, community-based consultations and do not form a significant part of the publicly funded healthcare system in the UK.

However, despite sporadic integration and high levels of private patient usage, many biomedical clinicians (particularly oncology surgeons and physicians) remain at best sceptical about the legitimacy of many CAM therapies and whether they should be provided to, or used by, NHS cancer patients (e.g. Baum, 2004). Doubts about the efficacy of CAM have deepened as EBM has become a central schema in healthcare planning and economic rationing in the UK (Pope, 2003; Sackett *et al.*, 2000). Although there exists a significant evidence-gap in relation to many biomedical cancer treatments (i.e. a lack of the high-level evidence for existing clinical practice), the EBM model is still consistently used rhetorically and practically as a means of justifying the limited provision of CAM within the NHS (Villanueva-Russell, 2005).

Doctors' views of CAM and patients who utilise it

It has previously been shown that oncology specialists may find certain issues difficult to discuss within medical consultations; prime examples being sexuality (e.g. Stead *et al.*, 2001) and death (Cherlin *et al.*, 2005). Similarly, there is some evidence that use of CAM is not discussed openly between cancer patients and their physicians and that CAM-related issues can create problematic dynamics within medical consultations (e.g. Adler and Fosket, 1999; Crock *et al.*, 1999; Mackenzie *et al.*, 1999; Tasaki *et al.*, 2002). The problematic nature of discussing CAM within the medical consultation is often, it would seem, reflected in silence rather than explicit or verbal conflict. Tasaki *et al.* (2002) reported three main reasons for patients' resistance to discussing CAM with their doctors: clinician indifference or opposition toward CAM use; clinician emphasis on scientific evidence; and patients' anticipation of a negative response from their clinician. In their study, some cancer patients reported physicians discouraging them from initiating or from continuing a discussion about CAM. Although useful, Tasaki *et al.*'s (2002) study did not examine a range of differently positioned clinicians' views (only physicians') and research is needed in other socio-medical contexts.

Survey research examining the self-reported attitudes of doctors to CAM has produced varied results, with some showing considerable support and others illustrating significant negativity. Astin *et al.* (1998) reported in their review of 25 surveys that roughly half of physicians believe in the value of at least one modality of CAM, most notably acupuncture, chiropractic and massage. In their study, Bernstein and Shuval (1997) found that, whilst nearly all of the physicians they interviewed would (or do) refer patients to CAM practitioners, in most cases the referrals were in response to patients' requests and did not necessarily reflect physician support for CAM. Other studies have illustrated the willingness of general practitioners to refer patients to certain CAMs (Goldszmidt *et al.*, 1995; A. White *et al.*, 1997).

It is worth noting that currently there exist no NHS guidelines on what advice medical specialists should give to patients who are using, or are interested in, CAM. National Palliative Care Guidelines for CAM have recently been developed for palliative care specialists, nurses, CAM therapists and allied health professionals in the UK (Tavares, 2003), but no such guidelines exist for hospital-based clinicians. There are some biomedical reviews of the use of CAM in medical oncology (e.g. Cassileth and Deng, 2004), but biomedical clinicians are often either unaware of the existence of such reviews or assume that if evidence was available for CAMs, individual treatments would receive high-profile exposure in biomedical journals.

Unsurprisingly, some doctors are thus uncertain as to what advice to give their cancer patients and how to respond to existing CAM use when it is reported in medical consultations (e.g. Adler and Fosket, 1999; Crock *et al.*, 1999). The situation is exacerbated by the fact that there is little agreement on what stance to take in terms of potential interactions between CAM and biomedical cancer treatments despite documented cases of potential interactions within the scientific literature (e.g. Weiger *et al.*, 2002).

Most importantly for this chapter, the research that has been done on oncology specialists' engagement with CAM has tended to focus on *their* own views of different therapeutic modalities and self-reported advice to cancer patients (e.g. Hann *et al.*, 2003). As such, there has been only limited research (i.e. Tasaki *et al.*, 2002) on how cancer patients themselves experience differently positioned clinicians' views of, and advice about, non-biomedical therapeutic options.

CAM and nursing

As outlined in the Introduction, the relationship between CAM and the nursing profession has historically been quite different from that of the medical profession. Nursing has frequently presented itself as patient centred rather than disease centred and holistic rather than mechanistic in approach. This, it could be argued, gives nursing practice something of a 'natural' affinity with some CAM approaches (Light, 1997) but also reflects some important differences between the trajectory or nursing and medicine (Boschma, 1994). CAM therapies like reiki, spiritual healing, reflexology, meditation or massage, on one level, may be seen to have broadly compatible objectives in terms of patient outcomes to that of nursing practice (e.g. reducing anxiety, stress, pain and discomfort). The emergence of CAM is thus potentially less challenging to the nursing profession than it is to certain elements of the medical profession.

This is perhaps best reflected in the increased levels of CAM advocacy within the nursing literature in the context of cancer care. There is significantly more support for integration and more research into the potential benefits of utilising CAM in conjunction with biomedical cancer treatments (e.g. Chong, 2006; Lengacher *et al.*, 2006). Moreover, at least within some facets of nursing, knowledge of (and the ability to offer advice on) CAM is represented as a valuable element to the cancer nurse's role in patient care (e.g. C. Lee, 2005).

On another level, certain sub-groups within nursing, it would seem, have begun to present the incorporation of CAM as a means of establishing inter- and intra-profession distinction (Tovey and Adams, 2003). CAM, in part, has thus emerged as a means of differentiation from the medical community (i.e. nursing as not merely a subsidiary of medicine) and within nursing itself (e.g. holistic or CAM specialties within nursing versus purely biomedical nurses).

Theoretical context

There has been considerable theorising about public perceptions of expert judgement and scientific knowledge in the social sciences in recent years (Beck, 1992; Giddens, 1991; Lupton, 1999). Beck's notion of reflexive modernisation has been used to conceptualise the (arguably) increased questioning of expertise within processes of (late) modernisation (Beck, 1992). The reflexive possibility of such a society means that people, it is argued, have become more sceptical about modern institutions such as science, no longer accepting at face value the judgements or advice of experts (Lupton and Tulloch, 2002) but, rather, actively assessing the merits of particular claims. This breakdown of certainties, such as belief in the all-knowing nature of the medical expert, has created a scenario whereby individuals (in this case cancer patients) are presented with a plurality of experts; a multiplicity of claims to truth that complicates an already difficult process of treatment decision-making. At first glance, this conceptual model fits well with patients attempting to balance biomedical oncological advice and knowledge with that espoused by different CAM modalities. The implication of the aforementioned arguments about this 'reflexive possibility' is that patients are forced to make active judgements about the veracity of particular claims and to engage critically with the merits of different ideological stances and knowledge frameworks. While the implication may be assumed to be a lessening of the authority of biomedical specialists, such an assumption has not hitherto been empirically tested in relation to CAM and cancer.

Moreover, at points of intersection in the context of a plurality of 'expert' advice (such as discussions about CAM in oncology consultations) processes of boundary work aimed at reinforcing territorial control may have a strong influence on patient disease and treatment trajectories. Whilst processes of boundary work have been regularly examined within the sociological literature in relation to CAM (e.g. Kelner *et al.*, 2004; Mizrachi *et al.*, 2005; Tovey and Adams, 2003), this has almost exclusively been focused on the methods by which different *occupational groups* (particularly biomedical stakeholders) have attempted to disrupt processes of CAM legitimisation and professionalisation. EBM, in particular, has been characterised as performing a normative function in medicine, regularly being used rhetorically and practically to justify limiting CAM integration (Broom and Tovey, 2007a). Such analyses have almost exclusively conceptualised the ideological and inter-professional struggle rather than how patients interface with (and negotiate) competing knowledge systems and forms of expertise.

Examining patient trajectories (and negotiation of expertise) is vital as such processes fundamentally impact on inter- and intra-professional dynamics and thus processes of boundary protection and disruption. The outcomes of, for example, discussions about CAM (as documented here) are fundamental in shaping patients' experiences but also bolstering/suppressing claims to legitimacy. The very act of engaging with biomedical clinicians about CAM potentially disrupts/reinforces the knowledge claims of different actors; it enters different ideological positionings and therapeutic practices into what has previously been largely a biomedical stage. Through an active engagement with CAM, patients contribute (albeit in a limited way) to the questioning of biomedical expertise.

As we outlined in the Introduction, such processes of lay critical engagement have been (albeit tentatively) linked to the so-called *deprofessionalisation* of medicine (see Haug, 1988), with such things as the Internet and CAM being viewed by some social commentators as contributing to a demystification of medical expertise and increasing lay scepticism about health professionals. The result, it is argued, is a decline in the power and status of the medical profession (Gray, 2002; Hardey, 1999; Haug, 1988). However, the question of whether patient engagement with CAM engenders (or is even contributing to) the deprofessionalisation of medicine is contentious and requires empirical investigation.

Practitioner responses to CAM use

Patients reported three distinct responses from their medical specialists regarding their CAM use or interest in using CAM – responses which had very specific impacts on patient action. These were: (1) explicit negativity; (2) supportive ambivalence; and (3) pragmatic acceptance. We identify broad patterns of correspondence between specialists' responses to CAM usage and patient action. Despite the theoretical possibility of a plurality of influences on patient action, oncologists' reactions to CAM (as perceived by individual patients) continue to play a significant role in influencing patients' decisions about the use of CAM therapies. Having recognised that, we should note that our intention is not to present a deterministic interpretation of outcome. Patients' accounts reflected an active engagement with decision-making on CAM (as seen, for instance, in their alliances with specialist nurses, discussed later). It should also be reiterated at this point that there exists a tension in this chapter between a focus on patient perception and the discussion of professional action. Our results are grounded in patient experience and perception rather than direct observation of therapeutic encounters.

Explicit and implicit negativity

Not surprisingly in view of long-reported antipathy amongst the medical community toward CAM, a strong theme that emerged from this study was that a significant proportion of the patients' specialists were either unsupportive or evasive in discussions regarding non-biomedical cancer treatments:

PARTICIPANT: Well, [specialist's name] was so very negative about anything that wasn't pharmaceutically led; I became very disillusioned with doctors, I'd say . . . he accepted nothing to do with nutrition at all. He said I could go out and eat McDonald's every day and it would have no effect on the cancer whatsoever. He said he was in charge of £5 million worth of cancer research money so he would know.

(male, English, 25 years, LP nodular Hodgkin's, metastatic)

Another respondent:

PARTICIPANT: When I have said I'm using these [complementary] therapies to my doctor he is just like that [shrugs his shoulders] . . . and that's it really.

(male, English, 81 years, prostate, metastatic)

Another respondent:

PARTICIPANT: Well, he just said, don't take anything, as it will interfere with your cancer treatment. You know, like prevent it working or something. Even though I knew [taking supplements] probably wouldn't hurt, I wasn't going to risk it so I stopped.

(female, English, 58 years, breast, undergoing potentially curative treatment)

Another respondent:

INTERVIEWER: Can you tell me about the dialogue with them in terms of what you said and what they did?

PARTICIPANT: They never admit that it's a good thing. They are not negative about it in saying it's a load of rubbish; however, what I find is that there is few little comments here and there just to bring things down that I don't like. I might be reading too much into but every time I mention [name of CAM practitioner], [name of medical specialist] at [name of hospital] says he just likes to put in that [name of CAM practitioner] is not registered as a medical doctor on the list of doctors, which I am sure he is because he prescribes things via a chemist and then [name of medical specialist] says, well, he might be just under a different name or I have spelt his name wrong or something like that, but he just puts these things in just every now and then.

INTERVIEWER: That's a slightly odd thing to say, isn't it, because either you're right, he either is a doctor or is not and he can either prescribe because he is a doctor or he can't prescribe, so its an odd thing to say, isn't it?

PARTICIPANT: Little things, little downer things.

INTERVIEWER: Why do you think he says that?

PARTICIPANT: I think he feels threatened by it because I say to him well aren't you interested in this oxygen therapies [sic], there are hundreds of books written on it, papers come out every year, and basically, no, he is not, he doesn't want to find out about it.

(male, English, 25 years, LP nodular Hodgkin's, metastatic)

These types of reactions from oncologists were consistently described as being alienating for patients and they reported 'closing up' and 'feeling bad' for even suggesting CAM use. The end result, amongst our respondents, of significant negativity within medical consultations was a strong tendency to avoid further discussion of CAM use with their oncologist. In turn, this resulted in a feeling of dissatisfaction with certain elements of the doctor/patient relationship and, moreover, a feeling of 'hiding things' from their specialist. This enhances patient anxiety, and, as one patient described it, 'was one more stress that I just didn't need'. In such cases there was a reduced likelihood of pursuing CAM unless other actors intervened (see the section on specialist nurses on pp. 88–92).

To add another layer of complexity, a common theme in these patients' accounts was how little time they actually get with their specialist and the importance of not 'wasting it' talking about 'non-essential' matters. Talking about CAM, it was suggested, could result in 'irritating them' and getting 'hurried out' of the office. Ultimately, a significant proportion of the patients we interviewed, after initial engagement with their specialist about CAM, if they did not drop the idea of CAM use altogether, opted to 'deal with' the CAM issue by themselves and not involve their specialist or GP.

In other cases patients reported that their specialist was not explicitly negative about CAM, but was either dismissive or noncommittal; such responses can also have a significant impact on patients' emotional wellbeing:

PARTICIPANT: I was having acupuncture, it was quite sort of . . . they were sort of dismissive I thought. They didn't actually ridicule it, but they said, hmmm [frowns]. I felt like they didn't really want to talk about it.
(female, Scottish, 70 years, breast, in remission)

Another respondent:

PARTICIPANT: They were noncommittal . . . they say they have no problem with it, which is very noncommittal . . . medics generally are so wary [about] people misinterpreting or quoting. I think what he was saying was he didn't think it would do any harm and it might do some good, that's how I interpreted it. I didn't push him much further.
INTERVIEWER: Had he said, 'Oh yes, here is a name of a CAM therapist,' would you have gone and done it?
PARTICIPANT: Yes, it would made a lot of difference, yes it would.
(female, English, 67 years, ovarian, metastatic, non-CAM user)

Even when oncologists were not particularly negative (as in the second excerpt), a lack of willingness to engage with the patient regarding potential CAM use was, in some ways, a passive form of professional gatekeeping. Being noncommittal was often interpreted by patients as oncologists not being willing to admit that they disapproved of patient action. Thus, it was assumed that whilst their specialists 'had no problem with it', it was best to avoid CAMs if possible, or indeed to avoid disclosing their use in the consultation.

Surprisingly, patients reported that junior doctors (i.e. registrars or house officers) were often much more negative than their specialist about CAM. This contradicts the argument that younger doctors are more open to patients' use of non-biomedical practices (Zollman and Vickers, 1999) and suggests the need for a reassessment of the notion that a more inclusive generation of doctors is gradually emerging.

Supportive ambivalence

The second broad response we observed in these patients' accounts of medical consultations was that of supportive ambivalence. This approach was characterised by the typical response of 'If it doesn't do you harm, it's probably OK'. Such responses were implicitly non-supportive of CAM but supportive of patient choice. Although this was reported to make patients feel like their oncologist did not want to engage with potential non-biomedical options, it had the advantage (over previous responses shown above) of largely not making patients feel like their CAM use was 'bad'. Moreover, it did not explicitly engender fear (through reference to potential harm or quackery) in order to push patients away from CAM:

PARTICIPANT: I asked the [specialist's name] and he said, 'If it makes you feel better by all means do it.' He said [the Gerson diet] just sounds like a generally healthy diet. But he also said there was nothing to suggest to him that it will beat cancer or stop the cancer returning . . . I think he said something like . . . there was no proof that it helped . . . he said something about, if it empowers you, if it makes you feel like you're doing something, then by all means go ahead. I think he looked at it from some psychological point of view rather than a medical point of view.

INTERVIEWER: How did you feel about that?

PARTICIPANT: It sounded like a vaguely negative thing to say but then I felt, well, it's my body, I'll do what I want with it.

(female, English, 28 years, breast, previously received potentially curative treatment).

Another respondent:

PARTICIPANT: My [doctor said], 'Be careful and don't get sucked into the religion, but I have no qualms about you doing it at all,' so he was quite willing. [Specialist's name] said, 'If you want to go for it, and you think it is doing you good, you go for it.' I mean I saw a different doctor and she said, 'Well, plenty of people try it.' She didn't commit herself. And I said, 'I think it is absolutely wonderful,' so she said, 'Well then, you know, you go for it.' . . . But they were all very wary.

(female, English, 56 years, Breast, metastatic)

As can be seen from the first excerpt above, although this ambivalent acceptance of CAM was not explicitly negative for patients there was often a patronising undertone within such response, with oncologists making it clear that patients were getting a placebo or psychological response from the particular CAM. Whilst not directly disapproving of patient CAM use, such discourses of 'placebo response' or 'psychological effect' implicitly undermined the legitimacy of the treatment and the philosophy of the particular modality. Moreover, according to the logic that informs this very discursive practice, making such statements potentially limits the very placebo they refer to:

PARTICIPANT: I remember talking to my oncologist once [about it and] he said, 'Well, whatever helps,' you know. But it is a bit like that, you know, it can't do any harm but, you know, they're thinking it can't do any good either . . . they tell you, you can't really do anything yourself to try and beat it . . . I wonder why they say that sometimes as it doesn't feel very good.

(female, English, 50 years, metastatic)

Whilst such responses may not be explicitly negative, they may serve to reinforce potentially undermining discursive representations of CAM, or indeed patient initiative and self-determination within disease and treatment processes. Doctors may be superficially 'nice about it' to patients but yet implicitly undermine their activities – an indirect but potent judgement in the eyes of many cancer patients. This, it would seem from the results here, merely enhances patient uncertainty and anxiety, and inevitably, as we shall illustrate later in this discussion, prompts patients to seek out other sources of advice about CAM (i.e. specialist cancer nurses). Again, therefore, we see that the responses of specialists to patient interest in CAM have (according to our respondents) a powerful influence on the way patients engage with therapeutic possibilities.

Pragmatic acceptance

In other cases these patients' specialists were highly supportive of patient choice, with patients reporting being encouraged to use CAM, and in a few cases even referred to CAM therapists for treatment:

INTERVIEWER: Can you talk about your consultant's approach to complementary therapies?
PARTICIPANT: He likes complementary therapies, does mine, one of my doctors, he is interested and he does put people forward for acupuncture and stuff like that, which not all doctors do that.

> (female, Irish, 69 years, bladder, previously
> received potentially curative treatment)

Another respondent:

PARTICIPANT: When I say to my consultant, 'Oh, I am doing ABCD,' he says, 'Oh well, between us it seems to be working, continue.' But he doesn't ask what, he doesn't go into that. I say, 'I am on diet and I do this and try and cut chemicals out and this that and the other,' and he will say, 'Oh right, well, whatever you are doing, it seems to be working so keep doing it.'

> (female, 60 years, breast, metastatic/remission)

These responses are indicative of the support some of these patients' specialists gave to their patients' use of CAM (albeit within a context of limited dialogue about paradigmatic issues) and the patients' own awareness of the difficult position that doctors are in. Reactions to patient interest in CAM were not all negative by any means and some of these patients' specialists made a concerted effort to assist their patients in pursuing non-biomedical options. A classic example of this was a specialist who persuaded the patient's GP to prescribe a homeopathic remedy on the NHS. Several such stories emerged where specialists could see the clear benefit resulting from a

CAM that the patient was pursuing and attempted to informally 'work the system' to assist patients.

Thus we have seen an interesting comparison of CAM use trajectories. Respondents in our sample with broadly similar levels of interest in CAM seemingly take forward very different forms of engagement with it. The approach of oncologists appears to be a pivotal (though not determining) factor in this. Oncologists act as gatekeepers at a practical level but also provide the stamp of legitimacy/illegitimacy at a discursive level, which patients continue to take very seriously.

Given the fact that oncologists are just one (albeit crucial) actor in the multidisciplinary cancer team, we were interested in contrasting their reactions to CAM with those of another crucial actor in the UK cancer services – the specialist cancer nurse.

Specialist cancer nurses as mediators between CAM and oncology

So what of the role of nursing in engaging with patients on CAM-related issues? Crucially, again, we need to ask both what the nature of their professional advice is and, indeed, how this impacts on patient action (bearing in mind the potential differences between views of doctors and nurses and the underlying status differential). We wanted to explore such questions as how do patients interpret specialist cancer nurses' views of CAM and how does this impact on treatment choices? Is there differentiation within oncology teams in terms of views of CAM, and clinicians' interactions with their patients? And if so, how do nurses manage such differences?

As an initial point of departure, we were interested in exploring these patients' perceptions of the relationship between nursing and CAM and potential collaborations. As it emerged within the interviews, the link between nursing and CAM was perceived as logical; something, as suggested earlier, of a natural progression from existing nursing practice and not paradigmatically problematic. However, there was notable differentiation in perspectives according to the 'type' of nurse being discussed:

INTERVIEWER: What do you think about the idea of nurses incorporating complementary therapies into their practice?
PARTICIPANT: I think it would be fairly logical step to take really if they have got skills and they can offer it and the patients are receptive or whatever. Just depends on the individual [nurse] I think. It would be a good thing.
(female, English, 42 years, sarcoma, undergoing potentially curative treatment)

Another respondent:

PARTICIPANT: [Some] nurses just come from the agency who are not really interested; they want to earn their money and I often think the nurses, the good nurses who are long there on the ward . . . they take [an] interest . . . you can see there are dedicated nurses and others who are just happy doing their eight-hour shifts or nine-hour shift without really bothered about looking [sic] . . . not being bothered about the patients.

(female, German, age unknown, breast, metastatic).

As can be seen from this, whilst these patients conceptualised CAM and nursing as not incompatible ideologically, there was also awareness of considerable differentiation within nursing (i.e. between specialists/non-specialists and permanent/temporary nurses), which in turn was seen to shape nurses' value within (and influence on) decision-making processes, and their 'suitability' to mediate between CAM and biomedicine on a range of different levels.

These patients' accounts also illustrated an informal system operating within these particular oncology settings whereby nurses would give 'advice' about nutrition and provide tips for reducing 'treatment side-effects' seemingly not espoused by oncology specialists:

PARTICIPANT: After having chemo the nurses do say certain things you can do but it's offhand. It's like, 'Drink lots of water' . . . 'Use this therapy' . . . and I am thinking, well, for what, one day, two days . . . again whether they can prove that or not, who knows . . . but that is what the nurses are saying [we should do] and it helps.

(female, Irish, 49 years, ovarian, metastatic)

This 'offhand' informal advice, although not always related to CAM or nutrition, facilitated communication about therapeutic options. Although these options may be 'unproven', such discussion was frequently noted by our respondents as being welcomed as an addition to their established biomedical treatment.

It also emerged in this study that specialist cancer nurses in particular (i.e. Macmillan nurses) play a very different and crucial role in supporting cancer patients' use of, or interest in, CAM. To provide some context, Macmillan nurses are highly trained specialist cancer nurses who provide support from the point of diagnosis. To qualify for status as a Macmillan nurse a clinician must have five years post-registration clinical experience, two of which must have been in cancer or palliative care. On top of this they must hold a degree in either palliative care or oncology. Most are specialists in a particular type of cancer (i.e. breast or lung cancer). As a result, Macmillan nurses have quite high status in oncology settings, which potentially influences their ability to support certain practices (CAMs) and mediate between patient perspectives and those of consultant oncologists.

In this study, Macmillan nurses in particular were consistently reported as suggesting 'safe' or 'valid' CAM options, often having a CAM therapist 'on their books' that they would send their patient to. Often this took place after the patient had had negative experiences in relation to discussing CAM with their medical specialist, and the Macmillan nurse played the role of 'damage controller'. Patients often reported sharing their negative experiences of interacting with their oncologist with their nurse and they would work out a strategy to incorporate both CAM and biomedical care into their treatment regime. In other cases, nurses would be the patient's first contact with CAM information and this would result in the patient trying out a CAM practice for the first time:

PARTICIPANT: On a recommendation of the Macmillan nurse . . . that's how I got to know about this [CAM centre].
INTERVIEWER: So have you used complementary therapies before that?
PARTICIPANT: I haven't, no, I didn't really know about them or anything. But I thought well if anything is going to work I will give it a go . . . and I trusted [name of Macmillan nurse].
(female, English, 47 years, uterine, curative treatment)

Another respondent:

PARTICIPANT: The Macmillan nurse who came to visit gave me two reiki names. She also sent me to [name of spiritual healer] at [hospital name] and I got on to other things through her and information I am being given by [other organisations].
(female, English, 60 years, breast, metastatic disease)

Another respondent:

PARTICIPANT: I got in touch with the Macmillan nurse when I was in hospital over Christmas, the other two or three other patients in particular were just urging me to . . . they were saying how much better they had felt for it and one was having, the one with the needles, you know . . . acupuncture, yes . . . and she [the Macmillan nurse] was strongly recommending that.
(female, English, 67 years, ovarian, metastatic)

Typically, patients would be sent by their oncologist to see a Macmillan nurse and the nurse would then advise them on all the different services they could use and suggest potential CAM therapies. The ones most regularly suggested were reiki, reflexology, massage, aromatherapy and spiritual healing (CAMs that, it could be argued, are more benign, less invasive and less paradigmatically problematic in relation to biomedicine). These nurses would give advice on CAM and discuss with patients the potential interactions between CAM and their biomedical care. Whereas the medical specialists would state that they did not know the risks, and therefore patients should probably avoid all CAM therapies that may pose a risk, the nurses would give specific information to patients on 'known interactions' and so on.

However, despite specialist cancer nurses' active engagement with CAM, and the important role that they seem to be playing in referring patients to

CAM services, these patients also reported an explicit emphasis (on the part of the nurses themselves) on the importance of recognising 'unproven' effects and on the fact that CAM treatments may not technically 'work':

PARTICIPANT: They [Macmillan nurses] said, 'No, in general we're not against [Traditional Chinese Medicine], we're not against it at all, but whether it does what it's supposed to do I don't know, but then nobody fully knows that.'

(female, English, 69 years, uterus)

Another respondent:

PARTICIPANT: The view [of the Macmillan nurses] was, 'Yes, won't do you any harm' . . . one of the Macmillan nurses, at Leeds, did say to me, 'I don't think it's a good idea to change your diet significantly.' So I suppose, don't do anything that you might consider to be extreme.

(female, English, 69 years, uterus)

Whilst advocating certain CAM approaches, the Macmillan nurses were also careful to reinforce the importance of biomedical measures of effectiveness, reminding patients that many CAM therapies were 'unproven' and that extreme regimes were 'unsafe'. Their gatekeeping of CAMs – directing patients to those they perceived to be 'harmless' – allows them to both maintain support and engage with patients but also warn patients off the more 'radical' therapies. In this sense, their engagement with CAM has the potential to shape what patients view as safe and appropriate in cancer care; a powerful form of gatekeeping.

Although nursing as a whole has divisions of opinion on CAM, in this case – with specialist cancer nurses – there was considerable homogeneity. What was evident in these patients' accounts was a perception of a generalised (biomedically referenced) support for CAM on the part of specialist cancer nurses. In terms of how this related to the views of oncologists, we might conceptualise this as primarily mirroring those specialists who maintained a 'pragmatic acceptance' approach, with the most negative nursing views never extending beyond those the oncologists maintaining a 'supportive ambivalence' approach. No experiences reported reflected the negativity of the first group of specialists discussed in this chapter.

As such there were two main consequences (in terms of patient action) of interaction with a specialist nurse about CAM. In the first scenario, dialogue about CAM was initiated with the specialist nurse and action was achieved – the nurse facilitated use of CAM. In the second scenario, the nurse acted as a 'mediating force', embarking on 'damage limitation' as a result of problematic encounters patients had experienced with their specialist. In such cases, as reported by some of the patients here, nurses acted to alleviate the anxiety produced by confusion or lack of dialogue about CAM within the medical consultation.

Within such processes these nurses have to carefully balance professional autonomy (providing independent advice) and biomedical dominance (their historical position of relative subordination within the biomedical hierarchy). The way in which they manage this dynamic may also be embedded in the specific character of the nurses in this study, i.e. the fact that they were senior, highly qualified specialised oncology practitioners. Their ability to operate largely independently from oncologists, and the degree to which patients accept their advice about CAM, will no doubt be, at least in part, mediated by this specific relatively high professional status.

Discussion

The aim of this study was to examine cancer patients' accounts of their clinicians' attitudes towards CAM and the ways in which dialogue within the patient/practitioner encounter shapes their perceptions of and usage of CAM. Specifically, we were interested in the range of oncologists' views encountered by patients; their apparent impact on action; and the role of specialist cancer nurses as a further source of professional input for patients. As with all research, our methods clearly impacted on the type of data collected, on our resulting interpretations and on the strengths and limitations of the study. Given the previous lack of attention to patient accounts in this area we felt it important that these should be central to this study. These, indeed, provided a hitherto unavailable insight into the phenomena under discussion. However, the focus on retrospective patient accounts meant an absence of direct observation of consultations. The next stage of research in this area should include such micro-level studies to examine and develop our findings.

As illustrated in the patients' accounts presented above, there were broadly three types of responses from medical specialists towards interest in or usage of CAM. Moreover, it would seem that the nature of an oncologist's response is influential in shaping decision-making about CAM. Specialist cancer nurses emerged as important figures – not least because of their mediating role between certain oncologists and patients.

The first type of response – *explicit or implicit negativity* – was experienced as highly alienating for the patients we interviewed, increasing their anxiety and invariably producing an unsatisfactory doctor/patient dynamic and thus decision-making process. Patients tended to react to such responses either by hiding their CAM use or by discontinuing it, regardless of the potential benefits they considered CAM to be providing. As suggested earlier, specialist cancer nurses often played the role of 'damage controller' in such cases, providing some redress to the negativity expressed by the patient's specialist, supporting existing CAM use and guiding patients towards what they considered the more 'appropriate' CAMs for cancer patients.

Supportive ambivalence – the second type of response we identified in the accounts of these patients – was not explicitly negative but allowed little in-depth dialogue about CAM. Moreover, such responses invariably involved the specialist denigrating CAM through the deployment of particular discursive representations. Such discursive practices tended to manifest rhetorically as 'inadvertent' comments about 'placebo response' or 'psychological effect' in relation to patients' suggestions of benefit from CAM. Such rhetorical practices were experienced as undermining and patronising, and, again, encouraged non-disclosure of CAM use within the consultation and in some cases diminished patients' enthusiasm for non-biomedical alternatives they were using in their own time.

The third response we identified was that of *pragmatic acceptance*. Such responses promoted a more patient-led open dialogue that allowed for discussion of both biomedical cancer care and non-biomedical therapeutics. In saying this, acknowledgement of a 'CAM effect' was almost exclusively a 'between you and me it's working' type of dialogue. Patients reported their specialists saying, 'Whatever it is, keep doing it,' in cases where they were clearly doing a lot better than anticipated. In such cases there was still very little dialogue about the paradigmatic basis of the therapy being used, but, rather, a mutual acknowledgement of its effectiveness and the legitimacy of the patient's decision to use it. Such positive responses tended to bolster these patients' determination to pursue non-biomedical practices and to enhance the doctor/patient relationship in terms of satisfaction with decision-making.

At some point in the decision-making and treatment process cancer patients are seen by a specialist cancer nurse, and, as it emerged in these interviews, there exists considerable differentiation between nursing and medicine when it comes to dialogue with cancer patients about CAM. This reinforces an emerging body of work in other disease contexts suggesting differentiation in how doctors and nurses engage with and mediate CAM (e.g. Tovey and Adams, 2002, 2003). Specifically, the results of this study suggest that nursing cancer specialists are enlisting (selected) CAMs as one element of their approach to patient care, providing advice and guidance regarding potential benefits and interactions, which CAM therapists to use and which CAM therapies are likely to be most 'effective'. This knowledge is, it would seem, largely experiential on the part of specialist cancer nurses but provides a valuable form of advice for patients regarding CAM. Broadly, the specialist cancer nurses maintained the pragmatic acceptance approach outlined in relation to the specialists, generally opting out of discussions about paradigmatic issues and focusing on patient-reported benefit and intuition to inform decision-making (rather than, say, the 'logic' of the treatment).

It is important to emphasise that this ability to provide CAM 'advice' and occupy a different position from that of many oncologists is likely to be embedded in the status of the specialist cancer nurse (and particularly the Macmillan nurse) in the NHS cancer services. Although further research is needed to explore such issues, it is probable that non-specialist nurses would be given less autonomy in what advice they provide to patients, and thus that CAM is in fact mediated by nurses differently according to their status relative to other nurses and biomedical practitioners.

The results presented in this chapter suggest that specialist cancer nurses are enlisting but also potentially transforming the nature of CAM by selecting out the 'best' therapists and the most 'appropriate' therapies for cancer patients. These 'CAMs of choice' were represented as the 'effective CAMs' and the 'qualified practitioners' as identified by the individual nurse. In playing this role, these specialist nurses effectively both enlist CAMs as part of their professional role and identity but also transform them by shaping patients' views of the CAM field and their pathways to CAM therapies.

Nurses also utilised discourses of potential harm (as well as benefit) in their gatekeeping with regard to CAM. There were regular accounts of nurses providing informal rules (i.e. not allowing CAM therapists to massage lymph nodes to reduce the chance of spread or not taking herbs that may interfere with chemotherapy) that are not actually backed up by evidence *per se*. However, such 'rules' were also reported as making patients feel like they are safe whilst enabling them to use selected CAMs. However, at another level this 'advice' from specialist nurses is also prescriptive, tending to lead patients towards the softer mind-based therapies rather than the whole-systems approaches like naturopathy and homeopathy. Thus, nursing is involved in CAM advocacy, to a degree, but is also contributing to the delimiting of CAM provision according to nurses own professional goals and belief systems. Specialist nurses, as gatekeepers and legitimisers of CAM, play an important role in shaping what cancer patients want from CAM, what they use it for and how they view it in relation to biomedical cancer care. This places specialist cancer nurses in a potentially powerful position in shaping the form of CAM integration in the NHS.

Whereas previously most work in this area has focused on inter-professional boundary work (e.g. Kelner *et al.*, 2004; Mizrachi *et al.*, 2005) and forms of intra-professional distinction (Tovey and Adams, 2003), what is suggested here is that crucial processes of gate-keeping or indeed challenge (delimitation and strategic promotion) also occur in grassroots clinical encounters. Moreover, these encounters and therapeutic relationships may play a fundamental role in influencing patient action and thus the reproduction, disruption and contestation of professional and therapeutic legitimacy. Moreover the intra-professional differentiation evident in the data further reinforces recent calls by sociologists to recognise the non-linear nature of the biomedical profession in ideological positioning and approaches to patient care (e.g. Broom, 2005; Timmermans and Kolker, 2004).

Given this diversity amongst practitioners and the active role played by patients in shaping action (as seen, for instance, in their alliance with nurses), what does this study tell us about the power of competing forms of expertise, and in particular the authority of medical specialists? Despite the potentially wide range of information sources and advice available to patients, and indeed the plurality of experts with competing claims of expertise and knowledge, this study highlights the fact that biomedical practitioners are still central to patient engagement with CAM. We are not, of course, arguing that one set of professionals determines the views and actions of patients; rather, that on the basis of these patients' accounts, medical specialists continue to hold a level of legitimate authority that is taken very seriously and has a discernible influence on patient action. This is important for an assessment of the value of conceptual arguments addressing the 'plurality of expertise' (outlined earlier) when attempting to understand processes surrounding CAM and cancer. While our results in no way undermine the notion of a generalised non-specific questioning of expertise (Lupton and Tulloch, 2002), and they certainly confirm the presence of competing sources of expertise (Giddens, 1991), both within and beyond biomedicine, they do not demand an interpretation which suggests a levelling out of the expert hierarchy (i.e. therapeutic pluralism) or the undermining of those with established power (i.e. a process of deprofessionalisation). In this case, at least, a multiplicity of 'expert' inputs does not necessarily bring with it meaningful authority for all of those 'experts', or a rejection of those experts grounded in 'science'.

This throws further doubt on social theory postulating a deprofessionalisation of biomedicine (Gray, 2002; Hardey, 1999; Haug, 1988), with significant ongoing patient reliance on biomedical expertise and judgement regardless of interest in, or usage of, CAM. Rather, it suggests a non-linear and partial restructuring on the part of biomedical stakeholders, with layers of actors who mediate CAM differently (i.e. nurses and specialists) and who have adapted to (rather than capitulated to) the increasing presence of CAM practices and therapeutic ideologies. This may in fact be more adequately conceptualised as a process of strategic adaptation (and, at points, translation), as oncologists and nursing cancer specialists respond to an evolving medico-cultural environment.

Finally, we should re-emphasise that this continuing centrality of biomedical specialists should not be taken to imply that patients were not actively engaging with the decision-making process. Whilst the influence of specialists' opinions was widely reported in patient accounts, there was also evidence of (limited) challenge to that expertise on occasion. Crucially, that challenge was more likely to be pursued where another source of biomedical expertise was available, relatively powerful and supportive. Where nurses' and patients' approaches exhibited commonality (and differentiation from those of an oncologist) specific forms of action were facilitated. In short, on the basis of this study we would argue that despite an apparent plurality of expertise surrounding the use of CAM in cancer care, cancer specialists remain the primary source of expertise and influence; any other expert influence was restricted to figures within biomedicine itself and even then that occurred in such a way that fundamental lines of authority remained intact. Competing claims to authority and expertise may exist; there is no evidence that in this arena they have significantly impacted on the legitimacy of biomedical experts.

5 Exploring the temporal dimension in cancer patients' experiences of non-biomedical therapeutics

Introduction

Methodologically and analytically speaking, research on patient experience of CAM has taken a 'snapshot' approach such as one-off qualitative interviews, focus groups or surveys (Cartwright, 2007; Sirois and Gick, 2002). There has been little or no examination of the potential evolution in patient experience over time and the influence of changing treatment and disease trajectories on perceptions of therapeutic options. Whilst in-depth interviews, focus groups and survey-based studies have provided crucial data for enhancing our understanding of user experiences of complex disease and treatment processes, there is still a distinct gap in our understanding of potential changes in experiences and perceptions over time and space.

In this chapter we utilise a solicited diary/unstructured interview approach, with its inherent ability to track experiences over time, to examine (1) the disciplining of the self demanded by certain CAM therapeutics and the impact of that on the experience of having cancer; (2) the role of CAM healing therapists in reconceptualising disease and filling perceived gaps in biomedical cancer care; and (3) the complex interplay between CAM-derived notions of self-healing and nearing death. The accounts examined here vividly illustrate the importance of day-to-day activities, patient/practitioner interactions and changing symptomatology (and lifespan) in patient experiences of CAM. We argue in this chapter that an emphasis on the temporality of cancer patients' CAM engagement is necessary to access a more nuanced understanding of the lived experiences of cancer patients. The findings also throw further doubt on conceptualisations of CAM use as engendering major paradigmatic cultural shift as indicated in much sociological work hitherto.

Empowerment, self-help and individual subjectivity

As illustrated in the previous chapters, the popularity of complementary and alternative medicine with cancer patients is considerable. Importantly, this so-called 'therapeutic turn' has been viewed by some social commentators as having considerable implications for healthcare practice (e.g. Mizrachi *et al.*,

2005), with the increased presence of CAM presenting a *potential* challenge to, and threatening the reconfiguration of, established biomedical organisational culture (e.g. Broom and Tovey, 2007; Coulter and Willis, 2004). Social theorists have made various attempts to conceptualise the implications of an increased therapeutic pluralism and a (seemingly) declining deference to biomedical expertise. Largely, conceptual debate has tended to espouse wider societal shifts, including those related to postmodernity, late modernity and new conceptions of wellbeing (e.g. Bakx, 1991; Doel and Segrott, 2003; Eastwood, 2000; Rayner and Easthope, 2001; Siahpush, 1998; Sointu, 2006; Tovey *et al.*, 2001). There has also been a significant body of work examining the role of CAM in individual experiences of disease. Within this body of work it has been posited that CAM may promote, for the individual, a number of things, including self-actualisation; empowerment or active roles; the reinsertion of subjectivity into disease and treatment processes; and a more rounded holistic approach to treatment (e.g. Bishop and Yardley, 2004; Burstein, 2000; Davidson *et al.*, 2005; McClean, 2005). Indeed, what CAM achieves for the individual patient has been of increasing interest to sociologists working in the area, who have produced a range of empirical and theoretical work (see also Broom and Tovey, 2007a).

However, the potential limitations of this 'therapeutic turn' beyond a purely biomedical approach, in terms of patient experience, have received little attention in the sociological literature. Moreover, in the context of cancer care and non-biomedical therapeutics, we know little about the day-to-day elements of the CAM experience and whether the paradigmatic shifts engendered in much CAM social theory are reflected in patients' lived experiences. In a wider political context of CAM promotion and advocacy amongst grassroots patient groups, political groups and the volunteer sector (Tovey *et al.*, 2007; House of Lords, 2000), the positive, empowering elements of CAM have been emphasised, with relatively little examination of struggle and complexity in CAM engagement. Indeed, whilst snapshot approaches to data collection have produced a plenitude of accounts of the CAM experience (e.g. Boon *et al.*, 1999), the mundane elements of the CAM journey have received virtually no attention in the sociological literature. The temporal nature of therapeutic engagement remains hitherto unexplored; specifically, how CAMs (and the discursive practices surrounding CAM therapeutics) are experienced, represented and reconstructed over time. To a great extent, the CAM experience has been viewed as largely static; as a persistent and concrete location rather than an evolving and changeable entity. The CAM user has tended to be conceptualised as making a permanent philosophical shift (i.e. toward individual wellbeing, regaining subjectivity and self-actualisation) rather than as an actor somewhat precariously positioned between a temporal world with multiple (and often competing) ontological and epistemological positionings. Particularly in the case of the cancer journey, this is a world in which positions of (ideological) dominance are *not* secured, but rather reinforced, contested and reconstructed over time and space (see Hall,

2005). Thus, in this chapter we ask the question: is there significant flux in the CAM users' perception, belief and everyday practice? Moreover, if there is, how would this disrupt (or indeed reinforce) previous conceptualisation of the CAM experience?

Therapeutic culture, self-help and disciplining the self

Reinserting the temporal dimension of disease (and CAM) experience necessarily involves a reconsideration of the theoretical (and, as outlined below, methodological) dimension. Beyond notions of self-actualisation and subjectification, what characterises the CAM trajectory conceptually in cancer care? The notions (and practices) underpinning much of CAM therapeutic culture – self-help, self-actualisation, wellbeing, subjectivity, individualisation, etc. – illustrate the positive, potentially liberating elements of the CAM experience. In fact, the sociology of CAM has largely been a paradigmatic critique of biomedical reductionism and positive epistemologies in general (see Broom and Tovey, 2007a). However, there is, we argue here, a need for a more balanced, critical view of the lived experience of CAM. The paradigmatic reconceptualisation of health engendered by widespread public support for CAM is accompanied by important changes in discourses of individual responsibility for (and practices around) self-health. In particular, the emergence of non-biomedical therapeutics may represent means of self-governance (above and beyond those related to CAM); virtual technologies of the self, one could argue, that promote a form of internalised (and potentially hegemonic) self-governance (see Foucault, 1988; also Armstrong, 2007).

It is here that Rose's (1999) work on governmentality and therapeutic culture more broadly is particularly useful (see also Rose, 2001). He suggests that in the second half of the twentieth century 'the very idea of health was reconfigured [to] encode an optimisation of one's corporeality to embrace a kind of overall well-being' (Rose, 2001: 17). This, he argues, has been amplified by self-help movements, therapeutic culture and alternative therapeutics which engender a 'working on the self' (Rose, 2001) as one element of good citizenship. Individuals, it has been argued, are thus colonised by discursive models of selfhood and agency that are not, strictly speaking, their own (Murray, 2007). At first sight, the emancipatory potential of self-health, self-help and new forms of selfhood seems sure; they are generally viewed as engendering the individual as the locus of decision and action, thus reinforcing the ideal of the liberal subject (Murray, 2007). Certainly, CAM has been conceived as a means by which subjects may be able to transcend or resist dominant biomedical conceptions of disease and bodily pathology. However, whilst there is no doubt a liberating element to certain CAM practices and ideologies (see Broom and Tovey, 2007a), do such representations accurately reflect all aspects of CAM engagement? As such, in this chapter we ask: can the processes and practices of self-healing espoused by CAM therapists (therapies) actually constrain, delimit or discipline the subject? Is there any value in viewing discourses (and the practice of) self-healing and wellbeing, as deployed in the context of CAM, as methods of self-governance, as technologies of the self that have potentially beneficial but also limiting effects for cancer patients. In order to capture the lived experience of the CAM user (and, indeed, to examine the relevance these conceptual concerns) an examination of the temporal dimension of illness experience is crucial. This necessarily involves utilisation of a methodological approach that captures how various processes, according to the individual subject, play out over time and space.

Diary methods

The use of diaries as a means of collecting data is by no means a new phenomenon (Elliott, 1997; Jones, 2000; Zimmerman and Wieder, 1977); however, their use has not been widespread, and in the context of research into CAM there has been no use of this methodology (Broom and Adams, 2007). Researcher journals have long been an accepted source of qualitative data for health research (Jacelon and Imperio, 2005; Jones, 2000; Smith, 1999) but there has been limited attention paid to the potential use of participant diaries or journals as a data-collection technique (Clayton and Thorne, 2000). This is despite acknowledgement in the literature that the diary–interview method, which combines solicited participant diaries and face-to-face follow-up interviews, can be used as an extremely effective method of data collection approximate to participant observation (Corti, 1993; Zimmerman and Wieder, 1977). As opposed to in-depth interviews or focus groups, the format of maintaining a solicited diary encourages participants to focus on daily activities and reflections that they value. Although diaries might lack the dialogical complexities and probing allowed in verbal communication (Begley, 1996), they also allow an examination of seemingly mundane day-to-day thoughts, processes and undulations; data that can be further explored in a subsequent interview (Elliott, 1997; Zimmerman and Wieder, 1977). This method of data collection has been used in feminist research to access the ordinary lives of women and to potentially transcend the *potential* artificiality and power dynamics of the face-to-face interview alone (see Hampsten, 1989).

A primary and significant benefit of personal diaries is the temporal nature of the insight they offer, allowing for flexibility and variation in the narratives presented (Meth, 2003). There is also some merit to viewing solicited diaries as an empowering tool for patients; indeed, all eight participants (one through his wife as he died before it was completed) commented that writing the diary was an extremely useful experience, providing a means of venting frustrations, recording emotional ups and downs and seeing 'the bigger picture'. Participants would also use them to monitor their condition and take a proactive approach. One respondent comments on the diary process below:

PARTICIPANT: I used the diary to test things out quite a lot and to document how often I went on the lymphasise; if I had an enema that day or something, what time I ate before I went to bed and what my night sweats were like. Because I was quite convinced that if I ate a lot close to going to bed that my night sweats would be worse, but now I don't think that's the case because it's all documented.

(male, 25 years, LP nodular Hodgkin's, metastatic)

Diary methods may actually provide a means, or indeed a different route, by which to express their emotions (Meth, 2003) and manage their treatment process, and thus, at least in part, can be considered an intervention as well as a method of seeking data.

Discipline in self-healing and remembering to be ill

A key theme that emerged from the patient diaries was the difficulty of maintaining motivation for non-biomedical therapeutic regimens over time. Waxing and waning of enthusiasm was evident in patients' accounts, and interactions with differently positioned clinicians (i.e. CAM therapists, nurses and doctors) emerged as influential in their therapeutic trajectories (see also Tovey and Broom, 2007). Whilst CAM (including rigorous diets, guided mediation, psychic surgery, herbs, vitamin supplements, etc.) was generally represented in a very positive light in the initial and subsequent interviews (i.e. as motivational and as giving hope), it was evident that such perceptions did not necessarily persist or remain static. As an example of this, in the following diary excerpts we see the day-to-day struggle of attempting to keep up enthusiasm for CAM and the crucial role encounters with biomedical and CAM clinicians play in driving or delimiting the ability of patients to maintain focus and enthusiasm:

Day 1: [The participant lists a substantial dietary and supplement regimen costing over £2000 a month, including daily caffeine enemas]. Although this seems like a lot to be taking it is fairly easy to regulate and really gives me the feeling like I am actively doing something every day. In addition to the pills I also try to do a coffee enema every day . . . I feel well in myself.

Day 2: I woke up feeling depressed today but after I went round to a friend's house and had a nice chat I felt much better. Then I received a phone call from [CAM practitioner], who told me he could see a definite improvement in my lymph. I went to bed feeling very positive.

Day 9: I am having a CT scan on the 17th of this month. I know that the results will look worse than my first CT scan. The doctors will stress upon me how important it is to have chemo. I do not want to hear how important it is to have chemo. I do not want to hear that as it will cast doubt and fear into my mind and it is important to stay positive . . . What a crazy world we try to live in.

Day 17: A CT scan at the hospital today. Spoke to the nurse, who was very supportive of my alternative approach. That's the kind of attitude I want from the doctors – not denouncing the unknown . . . it makes you doubt yourself . . . At the end of Yoga today I asked the instructor if there were any exercises I could do that stimulated lymph flow. He told me some. I told him why I wanted to do this and cried. When I got home I cried again, like when I first [had cancer] and had to tell people. It was nice to let go of some emotion.

Diary entries missing for a couple of days . . .

Day 24: Chatted with [my friend] today. I told [my friend] I found it difficult to keep motivated as I feel so well. Sometimes I have to remind myself that I'm ill, sometimes I slack off a bit for a few days, don't do enemas, don't lymphasise etc. . . . However, I do always take my supplements.

(male, 25 years, LP nodular Hodgkin's, metastatic)

A particular emphasis in the above diary entries, and those of the other participants, is the flux in motivation for CAM over time; a perhaps self-evident but also often understated aspect of CAM utilisation in cancer care. Ironically, sometimes the hardest moments – in terms of being 'self-disciplined' in maintaining a particular therapeutic approach (e.g. the Gerson diet)[1] – were when the participants felt well and happy with their lives. In such contexts there seemed to be an underlying tension between the need to 'heal oneself' through CAM and minimising how much time and 'headspace' it demanded. The day-to-day enactment of CAM seems riddled with personal (and highly individualised) struggle over not wanting to 'miss the good moments' (as a result of focusing too much on self-healing) but needing to be disciplined (remembering that 'healing' takes self-discipline). Certainly, in each of the diaries an element of self-disciplining was evident – an undertone that is likely linked to wider discourses of the self within therapeutic culture (Rose, 1999). These patients articulated in their dairies the need to 'think differently' about cancer, to seek 'self-healing' and minimise 'negativity'. However, the diaries showed that, whilst such notions could be useful at certain points for patients, they also formed a form of governance of the self; a process whereby patients felt bad if they 'slept in', 'missed an enema' or 'had negative thoughts'. Moreover, it would seem that, at least from the experiences of these patients, motivation for healing necessarily involves retaining a sense of pathology or 'unwellness' – an interesting paradox.

This has important implications for how we think about CAM sociologically. As a general rule, CAM practitioners do not focus on the terminality of disease or indeed biomedically conceived survival rates. Rather, there remains a focus on healing, self-actualisation or cleansing the body (see Tovey *et al.*, 2007). However, at least for these patients, the day-to-day act of 'doing CAM' necessarily involved *remembering* the root causes of their need for healing (and thus the presence of disease). This was accompanied by the sense that healing would *only* come through resolution (and comfort) with one's body and one's 'self'. Such an outcome, however, could only be achieved through taking a *disciplined* approach to self-healing (i.e. only eating organics, no milk products, no sugar, ensuring twice daily enemas, no alcohol and consistent meditation) and fully accepting an alternative conception of health, disease and the self. However, the reality of cancer care is that multiple ideologies are competing for the attention of the cancer patient and thus complete (and sustained) acceptance of one approach is at best difficult (see Broom and Tovey, 2007a). Thus, in such contexts pain or certain forms of suffering can be perceived as positive ('the chemo is having an effect') *and* negative ('I should feel better if the treatment is working') concurrently. This contradiction is particularly evident when combining CAM and biomedicine where patients seek 'healing' (i.e. symptom amelioration and wellbeing) but also want to 'blast the tumour' (i.e. tumour reduction) at the same time. The conflict between motivation coming from a need to 'feel well' and wellness as limiting motivation ('I just want to enjoy the time I have left') was a surprising and important theme in these diaries.

The impact of the practitioner was also evident in these diaries. As illustrated in the entries for Days 2 and 17 presented above, it was evident in each of the patient diaries how crucial differently positioned practitioners' perspectives were. A positive comment from a CAM practitioner or nurse to a CAM therapy seemed to drive motivation for days to come, and a negative reaction from a doctor tended to promote feelings of despondency and hopelessness. What was clear in the diaries was that clinician/patient interactions have significant flow-on effects for the days following the encounter. Moreover, each of the eight patients wrote about their interactions with biomedical clinicians about CAM; the majority of entries contained explicit negativity from medical specialists (see also Tovey and Broom, 2007) with considerable 'down periods' following such conversations:

> Day 26: Met with [medical specialist] at [hospital]. The CT showed a slight increase in some lymph nodes in my body. The meeting consisted of the same discussion/argument of chemo vs alternative therapies and nutrition. I asked if there was any chance at all of the NHS funding that part of my treatment. The answer was a definite no . . . he was very negative. I realise now there is no point in even discussing anything alternative with doctors. They are close minded and not willing to look into anything new unless it has been backed up with years of research in 100 patients or more. It would be very difficult to get these kinds of statistics since there is no funding . . . I get very angry at this.
>
> (male, 25 years, LP nodular Hodgkin's, metastatic)

The above respondent, and indeed, each of the other seven, reported similar negative reactions from their specialists and also periods of time after such conversations where their moods were low and their outlook became much more negative. As discussed elsewhere, the implications of an explicitly negative depiction of CAM can be quite serious (see Tovey and Broom, 2007). Given that these patients were all prolific CAM users – something each of their specialists was aware of – it would seem unlikely that a negative response would actually result in a clinician-perceived 'positive' outcome (i.e. patients stopping CAM use). As suggested by the above participant, it merely resulted in him withdrawing from discussion about alternatives to biomedicine, despite how important awareness of CAM use is from a cancer clinician's perspective (Zollman and Vickers, 1999). In each case patients described their psychological wellbeing being negatively affected by such encounters.

Friends dying, healing therapists and borrowed time

A key advantage of examining CAM experiences temporally is that we can gain insight into the more difficult periods in patients' disease and treatment processes and examine, in the context of each individual patients' approach, why these may be more challenging and potential methods of addressing emergent problems. It is worth noting that our research published elsewhere has suggested that the periods of time that cancer patients may find most difficult are those in between diagnostic and prognostic consultations; peri-treatment (when an outcome is not clear); and post-treatment (but before a formal assessment of treatment outcome) (see Broom and Tovey, forthcoming). What was interesting in these diaries was that certain CAM therapies (i.e. reiki, reflexology, spiritual healing, healing touch) seemed to fill in these 'spaces' of ambiguity and uncertainty, often calming patients down and reducing anxiety during waiting periods. Moreover, through conversations about disease and treatment processes, their healing therapists seemed to help patients reconceptualise their illness, providing 'alternative' conceptions of disease as not primarily pathological but rather innately human. Specifically, each of these patients (unsurprisingly) struggled to come to terms with the perceived terminality of cancer, often pondering what it means to live with 'a death sentence'. A key attraction of CAM therapists seemed to be the role they play in reconceptualising terminality and supporting patients through times in which they were confronted with the seeming inevitability of their illness. It was evident that CAM therapists (particularly those practising healing therapies) played a crucial day-to-day role in 'bringing them up' after setbacks and helping them get through the low points:

> Day 1: I have had a setback. I can be pretty positive about my illness most days but when you go for a scan it always makes you anxious. When you then have to go for further scans it really knocks you back . . .

> Day 2: I went to my reiki healer. My reiki healer is a wonderful man. I go there and I know that I will come from there feeling better. I spoke to him

and I told him my pain, he is so easy to talk to. I cannot talk to my family, it gets too emotional, they always say, 'You are strong, you will beat it.' He talked about how to heal myself, emotionally and physically.

Day 3: I do wish that some friends would discuss my illness but because I always try to put on a good front, I must give the impression I don't want to discuss it.

Day 7: Went for spiritual healing and much more relaxed. I always feel more at peace with myself when I have healing.

Days 11–16 omitted . . .

Day 21: Had a poor day today as one of the many friends I have made at the clinic has died. When one of your friends at the clinic dies it is very upsetting because you naturally think time is running out. You can do all things alternative and conventional but at times like this it brings home to you that you are living on borrowed time . . . but I know that I have to keep fighting.

Day 22: Feeling low. It was not my day to go for reiki but I felt I needed it and feel better. [Reiki healer] told me we are all on borrowed time.

(female, 66 years, breast, metastatic)

What we can see in the above entries is the crucial role reiki and spiritual healing – and the conversations that occurred within these healing sessions – played for this patient (and most of the other seven participants). Whilst trying to put on a 'brave face' for her family and friends, underneath she was extremely anxious and uncertain about how to make sense of her disease and prognosis. Her reiki healer calmed her down, normalised her mortality (i.e. stating that 'everyone is on borrowed time') and gave her a means of approaching her condition that was not orientated around cure rates or mortality. Again, in the interview following the diary stage she expressed this same sentiment:

PARTICIPANT: I think the bad days are because of this tiredness, I mean I just think to myself, God, is this as well as I am going to feel, you know? Like, I have always liked to go out visiting friends and things like that, and now, to be quite truthful, this past couple of weeks I could just sit in and, you know. Its not me, and I just think, well, am I on the downward slope? But then when I go to [reiki healer] and I come back I am rejuvenated. But, it doesn't last like it used to do.

(female, 66 years, breast, metastatic)

This important role was played (albeit to varying degrees) consistently by CAM (healing) therapists for each of the patients who completed the dairy in this study. Whilst simplistic notions of effectiveness, in terms of tumour reduction or symptom (pain or nausea) alleviation, may suggest these CAMs have only limited (or no) use, an examination of these patients' journeys and personal struggles (and existential crises) reveals key processes whereby CAM 'fills the voids' left in the context of biomedical cancer treatment.

However, as indicated above, a CAM-driven recontexualisation of disease (and the relationship of the self therein) may have its own implications (i.e. disciplinary effects), and indeed may be also hard to maintain over time. Whilst patients may be positive and upbeat about their condition in face-to-face interviews, the diary method gives us an insight into how emotions rollercoaster and into the volatile state that cancer patients may experience during disease and treatment processes. Events such as friends made at the oncology ward dying (as seen in Day 21 above) had a significant impact on these patients' overall wellbeing and ability to cope with disease and treatment processes. Seemingly peripheral events (a comment made at work about hair loss; a criticism of CAM by a biomedical clinician) had a dramatic impact on the lived experience of coping with cancer and so-called self-healing. Whilst the phrases 'thinking positive' and 'fighting hard' were used rhetorically in the interviews, the diaries illustrated the day-to-day struggle of maintaining a positive approach; death of friends or people they had come to know came as a hard reminder that patients were facing a difficult journey and a potentially shortened lifespan.

Nearing death and experiences of CAM

A strength of the temporal nature of our methodology and subsequent analysis was its ability to capture key moments of *transition* in these eight cancer patients' engagement with CAM and how their disease progression impacted on their preferences for and usage of CAM. Although we gave these patients a diary for only one month, even during this short period changes were evident in several of their approaches to CAM. Here we utilise the most extreme example amongst the eight patients who took part in this study to provide an indication of how patient experience of CAM *can* change dramatically near death. For this particular patient, the diary recorded his last month of life. Previously, he had pursued a rigorous dietary regimen called the Gerson diet, attending (costly) weekend meetings with his wife in CAM centres in cities other than where he lived (see excerpt below). At the time he was first interviewed for the first arm of this study, he and his wife were ardent supporters of the Gerson diet, spending hours a day preparing food and juicing in order to detoxify the body according to this treatment programme (i.e. 9 kilos of crushed fruit and vegetables a day, with hourly glasses of juice, in combination with three or four coffee enemas). As they were both in their eighties, this programme was very strenuous and was a huge commitment for both the patient and his wife. To give some context pre-diary stage, the following is an excerpt from the first interview completed as part of phase one:

PARTICIPANT: So we went [to the weekend retreat for cancer healing based on the Gerson diet]. I think eight of us were actual patients and three were supporters [of the therapy], so there were eleven of us altogether. They started off by us all having a meal together in the evening, and it was an organic meal and the chef cooked very well. The following day we had various sessions. First of all, talking to each other. They try to get you into a spirit of optimism that you will get over the problem and they said it's a mixture of physical, spiritual and mental messages that you can take to heal yourself . . . Well, I was well convinced that diet was very important . . . After we'd all exchanged our information, the director of the organization addressed us and told us how important it was to get into a mental state to improve yourself and they said that there would be. . . . can you remember the names? We received instructions on imagery . . . [The next day] we were asked to come down at 8 o'clock in the morning and do some exercises and these were breathing exercises and that's how you loosen up your limbs, but they did say that we had to think about being nurtured by nature. Forces that you can't measure, but they think there are forces in nature, which help healing if you can channel these forces into a positive line force. Being an engineer, you can't measure it so I'm at a loss to explain it.

(male, British, 82 years, lung, advanced)

The above excerpt provides an indication of the group they were attending in terms of ideological positioning and interpersonal dynamics. The diary begins at a time when the patient was becoming weaker and nearing death, with friends and clinicians concerned that the CAM treatments were too much. What follows is an emotional and difficult movement away from a rigorous diet, to a process of acceptance of death and an acknowledgement of finality:

Day 20: [Support group leader] came to see me after a session. I asked her why they were so against me using the Gerson therapy. She explained that it is a very demanding and time-consuming therapy and the clinic did not consider it wise at our age . . . This was a very valid point. I think that whilst I have made a critical change it will be best all round [to change to something else] and give us a quality of life together that Gerson could ruin.

Day 22: We have changed course to a less severe therapy therefore more suited to our age.

Admitted to hospital due to an infection . . .

Day 23: I'm awake at 4 a.m. I have resolved to attempt to modify my diet and exercise more as a self-help therapy. Life is difficult though now I'm on steroids and I don't know how to balance diet, rest, exercise . . . I am informed that a special bed will be delivered some time tonight to relieve my sores. I have been thinking of sitting in the chair all night with a blanket around me.

The above notes are the last he wrote in this diary. Four weeks later he died at 7.30 a.m. His wife delivered the diary and gave a follow-up interview.

(male, British, 82 years, lung, advanced)

The experience, and indeed difficulties, of utilising non-biomedical therapeutic approaches is vividly shown in this participant's last few weeks before he died. After pursuing a rigorous diet, this no longer became tenable as his condition worsened and he was then hospitalised. His support networks and family were hugely concerned about doing such a rigorous diet, and eventually he acknowledged this too. Such an example clearly raises the issue of just how tenable certain CAMs – and particularly regimens that take significant time, money and effort – may be at the end of life. Ideologies espousing individual healing (and undertones of self-responsibility as per those evident in therapeutic culture) put very specific demands on patients which have a very real potential downside for patients. Certainly, in the diaries and the subsequent interviews there emerged a potential guilt associated with 'not being disciplined enough' or 'not keeping positive'. The pressure to self-heal may actual prove problematic at different stages of disease and treatment processes (particularly at the end of life). Moreover, developing a better understanding of the pressure patients impose on themselves in relation to healing will assist in providing more effectively for the supportive needs of patients at key points of transition.

Discussion

In this chapter we have provided the first examination of cancer patients' experiences of CAM using a solicited diary/unstructured interview approach. In so doing our aim was to build on existing work which has provided a snapshot of patients' engagement with CAM to begin to work towards an understanding of evolution of time and the sense of the fluidity which is integral to that process.

By using diaries (with their inherently temporal nature) for the first time in the analysis of CAM use by cancer patients, this study has drawn attention to several key issues that cancer patients face which have not hitherto been highlighted in the sociological literature. First, there is a tension in CAM users' experiences of cancer between the need to 'heal oneself' through CAM and minimising how much time and 'headspace' this demands. An underlying theme of self-responsibility (often reflected on as 'needing to be disciplined') was prevalent in their written accounts, with, ironically, 'feeling well' presenting as a problem in keeping up motivation for CAM use. As such, the CAM experience, at least for these eight patients, seems to have paradoxical effects. It engenders, on the one hand, a liberation or emancipation from restrictive prognostic biomedical data (i.e. through the promotion of notions of self-healing, self-actualisation and wellbeing rather than cure and terminality), whilst, on the other, *also* promoting a need for discipline and self-responsibility (i.e. 'I need a *more* rigorous diet' or 'I need to be *more* positive'). Whilst CAM-derived individuation and subjectification (see Broom and Tovey, 2007a) may provide some amelioration from biomedical prognostic (un)certainties, it may also, it would seem, pose other subtle but important difficulties for cancer patients.

It should be emphasised that we are not arguing that this is necessarily a pathological facet (or failing) of CAM; rather, it points to the fact that more attention should be paid to the power dynamics (and disciplinary effects) inherent in non-biomedical therapeutics. Moreover, there is a need for consideration as to how self-help and new conceptions of disease and selfhood may actually facilitate a governing of the subject. Conceptually the flip side of so-called subjectification and individualised conceptions of the self (in tandem with wider discourses and self-help and wellbeing) may actually constrain the subject (Rose, 1999), creating dilemmas between self-actualisation and empowerment and self-responsibility and disciplinary effects (Foucault, 1988).

The day-to-day changes in mood and anxiety directly shaped patients' ability to enact CAM; moreover, such changes were directly related to the input from a range of differently positioned practitioners (both CAM and biomedical). As shown by the authors elsewhere (Tovey and Broom, 2007), input from clinicians plays a quintessential role in influencing patient wellbeing and psychological state. Diary entries revealed the variation, the ebb and flow, of individuals' relationship with therapeutic options. They highlighted the limitations of, for instance, attempting to understand the motivation of 'users' versus 'non-users' at a single point in time.

The complexity and non-linear nature of the CAM experience emerged as we saw the powerful and positive role played by *certain* CAMs in these patients' disease and treatment trajectories. Healing therapists, in particular, seemed to fill the gaps evident in biomedical cancer care, helping each of these patients in times of ambiguity and uncertainty and providing alternative conceptions of disease during the often drawn-out process of receiving biomedical cancer care. The supportive needs of patients with cancer are often sidelined in order to ensure cure rates are maximised (J. Turner *et al.*, 2005); CAM practitioners, and particularly those in the healing modalities such as reiki, reflexology and spiritual healing, may provide a crucial service which addresses the psychosocial needs of some cancer patients (see Broom and Tovey, 2007a). Existential crises are common during times of cancer diagnosis and treatment, and biomedical cancer clinicians may not always have the time (or intellectual resources) to deal with such issues; it would seem that healing therapies could play a key role in this context. The key difference, in terms of experiences of CAM engagement, may lie in the overall objectives of the therapy; whilst the dietary regimens (e.g. Gerson diet) and other whole-system CAMs (i.e. naturopathic or herbal regimens) promote 'self-healing' and help in 'fighting cancer', the healing therapies (and therapists) tend to focus on amelioration of symptoms and easing anxiety and stress over fears of pain and terminality.

Although further exploration is needed (i.e. different cultural contexts with larger sample sizes and a broader range of disease and treatment types), we suggest from these results that the ability to 'do CAM' (and faith in CAM logics of self-healing) may shift dramatically when nearing death. Moreover, it is possible that the notions espoused by many CAM practitioners (i.e. healing, self-help, wellbeing and self-awareness) may actually make the transition quite difficult for some individuals. The notion of 'healing oneself' through diet, meditation and self-discipline may in fact be hard to let go of as disease progresses and the more rigorous CAM therapies become unrealistic. Moreover, how patients reconcile 'success' when they get to an advanced stage (i.e. 'Have I done enough?'; 'Maybe I wasn't positive enough') warrants further investigation.

So how does the temporal dimension of the CAM experience fit with previous conceptualisations of CAM? Ultimately, previous social theory as applied to CAM has, perhaps inadvertently, produced a rather static and unchanging illness experience. It has focused on a paradigmatic shift in cultural values (i.e. shifts to postmodernity; individuation) (e.g. Bakx, 1991; Doel and Segrott, 2003; Eastwood, 2000; Rayner and Easthope, 2001; Siahpush, 1998) rather than a focus on individual illness experience and the fluidity of perception and experience in day-to-day life within disease and treatment processes. We argue here for a re-examination of how individual experiences shift and flow; how representation (and experience) may change over time and as disease progresses. Ultimately, we argue for a sociology of CAM which examines the day-to-day (seemingly mundane) experiences of 'being CAM users', incorporating the uncertainties, changeability and ambiguities inherent in the cancer journey.

6 The problematic nature of conflating use and advocacy in CAM integration

Introduction

The notion of 'integrative medicine' has been hotly debated in the medical literature over the last decade (e.g. Caspi *et al.*, 2000; Ernst, 2005a). However, there still exists little or no consensus on what *integration* actually means in oncology contexts, or, indeed, on the most effective means of achieving 'an integrative approach' to cancer care. Much of the debate about integration in cancer care has centred on evidence production and the degree to which CAM therapies can be justified in a UK policy context espousing evidence-based practice (Ernst, 2005a). Regardless of such debates, pockets of grass-roots integration are becoming more evident in the UK, particularly in the context of palliative and hospice care (Broom and Tovey, 2007). However, little empirical attention has been given to how attempts at integration are actually regarded by cancer patients.

The work which has been done in the area of CAM and cancer has focused on what cancer clinicians and other biomedical stakeholders think of actual or potential integration (e.g. Hewson *et al.*, 2006). As a consequence a tendency to conflate use of CAM services with support for the process of integration into state-funded services has emerged (e.g. Frenkel and Borkan, 2003). It is regularly assumed that the majority of cancer patients' view CAM integration as *prima facie* good. However, this assumption has little empirical evidence to back it up. While high levels of personal usage amongst cancer patients (see Cassileth and Vickers, 2005) *may* translate into widespread support for integration into public-service delivery, this cannot be treated as inevitable. To date, we know little about cancer patients' views of the benefits and limitations of integration; the relative importance of evidence in driving integration; the relationship between financial cost versus physiological (and psychological) benefit; and, finally, the importance of the context of delivery (i.e. location/provider type) on experiences of integrative care.

The aim of this chapter is to examine empirically this assumption of cancer patients' support for CAM integration. In so doing we argue: (1) that a characterisation of unequivocal cancer patient support for integration (even amongst those who use CAM) is an oversimplification and distortion of the situation; (2) that it is inappropriate to conflate 'use' with 'advocacy'; (3) that patients' engagement with the idea of integration is complex and multi-layered; and (4) that this complexity can be explicated by looking at key dimensions of an integrative process – evidence and risk, cost and provider legitimacy.

Background

There has been much debate about the potential benefits and pitfalls of integrating complementary and alternative medicines into the NHS cancer services (House of Lords, 2000). Although there is already sporadic integration, CAM is not provided on a systematic basis to NHS cancer patients despite substantial private usage. In May 2006 the Foundation for Integrated Medicine (2006) presented findings from a report commissioned by the Prince of Wales, arguing for greater momentum toward the integration of CAM into the NHS. This was strongly rejected by prominent members of the British medical establishment, who promptly called for any existing funding of CAM (however limited) to be discontinued (Baum, 2006) in a very public denigration of CAM. Despite the more consensus-driven approach of the last decade, integration remains a contentious issue amongst practitioners and policymakers.

It is useful, for the purpose of providing a background to the results presented in the next section, to outline some of the key issues in such debates about integration. In particular, we focus here on those related to: (1) evidence of effectiveness; (2) risk of harm; (3) cost effectiveness; and (4) provider legitimacy.

Integration and evidence

The most prominent debate regarding CAM integration has been over evidence of effectiveness and the need to adhere to the basic tenets of evidence-based practice. It is commonly argued that CAMs have little high-level evidence to back them up in terms of cancer care and thus should not receive NHS funding, although it is not entirely irrelevant that many biomedical cancer treatments lack this very high-level evidence (Broom and Tovey, 2007). Regardless, debate continues on the degree to which CAM modalities are backed up by biomedical-type evidence.

Despite the common perception, and as suggested previously in Chapters 1 and 3, there is in fact some evidence of effectiveness for certain CAMs for cancer care. RCTs have shown that acupuncture and acupressure are practical, safe and inexpensive ways of reducing nausea and vomiting after cancer treatment (e.g. Ernst, 2001; Filshie, 1990). Forms of healing (e.g. reiki and therapeutic touch) and mindfulness-based stress reduction have also been shown in clinical trials to lower anxiety, enhance quality of life and improve overall wellbeing in cancer patients (see Carlson *et al.*, 2004; Ernst, 2001;

Tavares, 2003). However, other CAM therapies provided by some NHS organisations, such as aromatherapy, massage and reflexology, have little high-level biomedical evidence to back up their efficacy in cancer care (Corner *et al.*, 1995; Soden *et al.*, 2004; Stephenson *et al.*, 2000).

Biomedical cancer treatments are currently *more* evidence based than most CAMs (Broom and Tovey, 2007). However, inevitably such debates about evidence have led to questions about the measurement of treatment effect; trial design and implementation; and the problems associated with complex interventions. Most biomedical interventions are well suited to their existing methodological processes and thus have little to gain from methodological restructuring. Varying degrees of publication bias also mean that biomedical journals may be more likely to publish negative findings for CAM interventions. In addition, CAM interventions are more likely to be tested and published in non-English contexts (Pham *et al.*, 2005). Moreover, as highlighted in Chapter 1, little attention has been given in debates about evidence to how cancer patients themselves assess effectiveness and the degree to which they view an evidence base as necessary for integration (or as a justifiable means of excluding CAM therapies).

Integration and risk of harm

Risk of harm associated with use of CAM by cancer patients is an area of concern to both clinicians and patients. It is not uncommon for patients to assume that CAMs are largely benign and pose no significant risks to cancer patients. This assumption has been shown to be inaccurate (e.g. Ernst, 2002; Ernst, 2005; Pittler and Ernst, 2003). There is, for example, evidence in the biomedical literature of interactions between selected CAMs and biomedical cancer treatments (Weiger *et al.*, 2002). The exclusion of CAM from patient care can thereby be justified, some would argue, purely on a lack of evidence of safety, regardless of evidence of effectiveness. However, risk is a complex issue and is quite subjective for the individual patient. Exactly what level of risk is acceptable is not easily quantifiable. In biomedical treatment, risk is generally assessed relative to quantifiable benefit as evidenced in RCTs. If, for example, intensive chemotherapy gives an 80 per cent improvement in five-year survival, but increases the chances of developing leukaemia tenfold, a medical specialist may still argue that this is a reasonable risk/benefit ratio. Clinicians are regularly faced with risk/benefit ratios like this, but yet assessment is highly subjective for the individual patient. Such problems are compounded when, as is often the case with CAMs, benefit is also disputed. In such cases, even very small, anecdotal risks related to CAM can be used to rationalise their exclusion (Broom and Tovey, 2007). It is also the case that some commonly used CAMs offer virtually no risk (e.g. reflexology, reiki and aromatherapy), indicating the need for a nuanced approach to assessing the merits of integration.

Cost effectiveness

Estimates of the cost effectiveness of CAMs are infrequent if not non-existent for many interventions. In the case of cancer care they are virtually non-existent, and indeed issues related to cost effectiveness become more ambiguous in this disease context (i.e. whether perceived alleviation of symptomology is 'cost effective'). Canter *et al.* (2005) found that use of a number of evidence-based CAMs for a range of health problems (not related to cancer) was actually more expensive than the usual (biomedical) care; moreover, they found that the outcomes may also not have been as good for the patients (the treatments were still effective, but not as effective as the usual care). Of course, in the context of cancer care notions of cost effectiveness become complicated by the emotive nature of the disease and public support for the alleviation of suffering by any means possible (regardless of, say, documented quantifiable treatment effect). Thus, the question of cost effectiveness is transformed into the question: does it benefit the patient enough to warrant funding?

From the limited research available, what we do know is that even when patients are given the choice, it is likely that actual costs for alternative services compared with those associated with biomedical cancer care will be extremely low – less than 2 per cent in a group of insured cancer patients in the US (Lafferty *et al.*, 2004). Moreover, relatively cheap interventions may have a significant impact on patient satisfaction with care (e.g. Milligan *et al.*, 2002) and lower usage of biomedical pharmaceuticals.

Provider type and context

There is considerable debate about who should provide CAM to cancer patients, if indeed integration is to occur, including the roles of nurses, allied health professionals and CAM therapists in such provision (e.g. Frisch, 2001). Such issues are far from clear cut, with arguments about the watering down of CAM ideology and clinical expertise when provided by non-CAM clinicians (i.e. with limited training in CAM interventions). There are also arguments about the advantages of using nurses with existing therapeutic knowledge to ensure the 'safety' of CAM delivery. However, the significant CAM advocacy within certain elements of the nursing profession (e.g. Chong, 2006; Lengacher *et al.*, 2006) has been viewed by some as the expropriation of CAM by nurses. As seen in the current study, in NHS settings where CAMs are provided nurses are often placed in coordinating roles. CAM advocates often argue that such processes of the enlistment of CAMs (and, in actuality, their translation) (see Broom and Tovey, 2007) merely function to water down ideology, biomedicalising CAM rather than providing integrative holistic cancer care (i.e. integrating both CAM and biomedicine). However, there has been no research on what cancer patients actually prefer and for what reasons.

The context of provision is also related to this point. As yet there has been no research on the importance of setting on experiences of CAM. We know virtually nothing about experiences of hospital-based CAM therapies versus those within the community.

Cancer patients' perspectives on CAM integration

In looking to unpack patient perspectives on the integration of CAM into state-funded cancer care we need to consider both how respondents discussed the issue at the broad level of principle and how they engaged with the issue when given the opportunity to look at the practical application of an integrative policy. As will be seen, while initially the use–advocacy link appears to be in evidence, once an examination of those building blocks of integration (evidence and risk, cost and practitioner legitimacy) are considered it becomes clear that a more sophisticated interpretation of the situation is required.

Our first task was to get a sense of our respondents' initial feelings about the merits of integration – a sense of their baseline assessment of the issue.

PARTICIPANT: I do think [integration] is a good idea.

INTERVIEWER: Specifically for cancer patients?

PARTICIPANT: Yes, I do think, because, it just gives . . . but I think it makes you positive, it does make you feel positive, because, like I say, it just takes you away from all the horribleness of the cancer just for a period of time. I think that if that is the case, then it's got to be a plus point for you because it makes you feel better.

(female, British, 33 years, malignant melanoma)

Another respondent:

PARTICIPANT: For cancer patients, then, I think yes. I think anything that makes a person feel cared for, looked after and not as frightened. I mean you only have got to look at hospices, haven't you, for a start off? They do anything like that for people who are dying of cancer. They give them any kind of alternative therapies and people die in these places, not *happy* exactly, but very much different from dying in an ordinary hospital or dying at home.

(female, English, 59 years, vulva)

Another respondent:

PARTICIPANT: I think that complementary therapies, they're such a benefit. Not just for the patient but they could be to the whole family. And when they saw that their mother, father or husband or wife was coping better, it would make it easier to care for them. And it would be so good for the patient themselves. I think it would be a wonderful thing personally. A wonderful thing to offer it.

(female, Scottish, 70 years, ovarian)

As can be seen from the above quotations, on this initial level – and when it was initially discussed in the interview – the majority of the patients interviewed here supported the fundamental notion of integrating CAM into the UK cancer services. In this preliminary discussion respondents tended to focus on the therapies themselves, on their intrinsic benefits, rather than on issues relating to how integration might occur and what the broader implications of that might be. Respondent focus was on the identification of a set of therapies which were considered of value in the management of cancer. At the beginning of each interview, most participants maintained a 'whatever makes people feel better' approach to CAM integration. Cancer patients, it was often argued, should be given *any* support or intervention that might help them through such a difficult time. In isolation, such comments could be viewed as evidence of cancer patients' overwhelming support for CAM and integration, but, as illustrated below, when discussed in more depth, the concept of integration becomes much more complex and differentiated. In actually, such questions as what will be provided, what will it mean for wider health provision and who will deliver it are fundamental to patients' perceptions of the legitimacy of integration. As the interviews continued, the complexities of what integration actually means (e.g. ideologically and economically) ultimately came to the fore.

Evidence and risk

As suggested previously, debates over evidence have dominated the inter-professional dynamics between CAM and biomedicine. In the context of cancer care, where emotions tend to run high, such debates has been particularly heated, with huge inter- and intra-professional divisions over what constitutes evidence and how it should be applied in clinical practice (Broom and Tovey, 2007). Given this background, we explored the importance of evidence for integration with our interviewees. What we found was that patients applied very different standards to their own decision-making compared with those which they felt should be applied when considering the systematic integration of CAM into the NHS. In the main, patients considered scientific evidence to be unnecessary for their own decision-making but necessary to justify NHS funding. This is a finding which immediately brings into question the validity of any assumption that use, in itself, should be taken as an indicator of a simplistic support for integration:

INTERVIEWER: Do you think we need proof before [complementary therapies] can be integrated?

PARTICIPANT: Well, I don't need proof because I am quite happy, you probably get people that are having it or have had complementary therapies that would agree [to integration], but these other people, the people that are going to fund it in the NHS, I think it would be them that you have got to argue with. 'Should we be spending the money

somewhere else?', that's what I think the argument is . . . so, yes, we need
evidence.

(female, English, 48 years, leukaemia)

Another respondent:

INTERVIEWER: How do you decide what should be provided and what
shouldn't?

PARTICIPANT: That's the thing, I suppose, for more research to see . . . and
there needs to be more research on specific therapies to see if people can
[get benefit]. Again, it's difficult to articulate the benefits [of complementary therapies], so it does prove very difficult, but I suppose we need
to look at people who have undergone or have started taking specific
therapies to see what specific benefits they got from those therapies.

(female, English, 31 years, non-Hodgkin's lymphoma)

There was thus a distinct ambiguity around the role that evidence should
play in decisions about integration. This was centred both on existing
bureaucracies, and the need to appease them, and on the nature of the individual therapy being considered. There was an underlying sense that one was
not going to be able to change the trajectory toward EBP and a resignation to
the fact that evidence was necessary and inevitable to underpin structural
change; it was just not deemed to be important personally. For the individual,
experimentation and/or experiential knowledge were frequently presented as
a valid basis for action.

However, views on the need for scientific evidence were also mediated by
the nature of the individual CAM therapy being discussed. What we found
was significant variation in patient perspectives, with a split between the
importance of evidence according to what one might call the 'whole-systems
CAMs' (e.g. homeopathy, naturopathy or specific dietary regimes) and the
healing-based therapies (e.g. reiki or spiritual healing):

PARTICIPANT: I think [reflexology and healing] are fine. Complementary
medicines or complementary therapies which are not medicinal, I have
no argument with at all. It's the medicinal ones that need, well, they all
need to be tried and tested. We don't want anybody doing damage with
sort of physical alternative therapy because it isn't tried and tested. With
medicinal I think is a bit more crucial that methods are tried and tested.

INTERVIEWER: Why do you think that it is more crucial?

PARTICIPANT: Well because it gets into your system, doesn't it? You could be
poisoning yourself, couldn't you, if it's not tested? I mean it might do
good to one part of your body but might do harm to another part.

(female, English, 66 years, breast)

This perspective was common amongst these patients, with a general distinction being made between 'internal' and 'external' CAMs. Those which were

'inside' or 'consumed' were viewed very differently from those that were external or psychotherapeutic. In the case of ingested substances, harm was viewed as much more significant an issue, and the solution: evidence production. The majority of patients considered it fair that ingested CAMs prove their worth before receiving funding or legitimacy in the NHS. Thus, we see not only that patients are prepared to raise the issue of evidence as the basis for integration, but also that they frequently do so in a way which incorporates a subjective assessment of the varying levels of risk associated with the use of particular modalities. Avoidance of harm was as pivotal as the measurement of benefit.

As well as differentiation in perspective according to method of application (i.e. ingested versus experienced; internal versus external), a strong underlying issue in such accounts was perceptions regarding the aims or objectives of certain CAMs. Whereas the 'whole-systems' approaches were perceived to be aiming at cure or physiological improvement, healing modalities were viewed as psychotherapeutic in their approach and objectives. Thus, the need for evidence was mediated by the objectives of the modality and its therapists. As such, perceptions of the importance of evidence are non-linear and deeply embedded in the nature of claims-making and therapeutic process. Moreover, the need for scientific evidence was often also mediated by a sense that the NHS was overstretched and that any further burden might be 'the straw the breaks the camel's back', as one respondent stated. With that in mind, we now move to the issue of economics.

The economic costs of integration

As will now be shown, views on the costs of integration again reflected the diversity and complexity that was evident with the themes discussed above. There was no simple association between use and a positive assessment of the costs involved in greater funding for CAM within state-funded services. A significant proportion of patients (it should be re-emphasised that the overwhelming majority of these patients were CAM users) felt that CAMs were not an extra cost that the NHS could cope with and thus considered integration to be problematic at best. However, others viewed CAMs as minimising reliance on biomedical pharmaceuticals and thus compensating for their cost to the NHS:

INTERVIEWER: How do you balance cost, as in money, with benefit?
PARTICIPANT: Me personally, I don't mind the cost. I would like the benefit and I am quite prepared to pay as much as I can afford for things like that ... but I certainly don't expect the NHS to fork out for ... it would be nice if they could but I don't think they can afford it. There is a limit and you have to be fair, there are very poorly children and they need their treatment first.

(female, Irish, 68 years, bladder)

Another respondent:

PARTICIPANT: Yeah, there's more and more people needing the [biomedical cancer] services and I know drugs aren't cheap. And I think the cancer care now is marvellous but you've got to think where your priorities are. I mean, even though I think [complementary medicine] is absolutely fantastic, could the national health afford it? Which I don't think they'd be able to and I think if people want to do it, if the information is there, they will do it. I mean if the national health did it, would it only be for cancer or would it be for people with other things? You don't know because you start something small off like that and everybody gets on the bandwagon, don't they?

(female English, 56 years, ovarian)

PARTICIPANT: I am not taking painkillers so therefore I am saving the NHS this money on painkillers so why shouldn't they put it onto something else? So much money is wasted in the NHS, why not? I am in a fortunate position that I can afford this £20. There will be some people who would love to go for it but just cannot get £20 . . . When I think how much good it does me, why shouldn't everybody have access to this? Now, how much are painkillers? I mean, people are shoving painkillers in like sweeties . . . now I don't know how much morphine costs, but if she'd go for reiki she probably wouldn't need as much morphine . . . if I wasn't going for reiki and other complementary therapies I would be taking painkiller tablets, so why shouldn't they be willing to give you it on something that is doing you good?

(female, English, 51 years, bowel)

As can be seen from the above excerpts, even amongst this group of predominantly CAM users there was considerable differentiation in our respondents' views of the economics of providing CAM. What emerged was a clear split between those who did not consider cost a consideration in the context of cancer care and others who found it difficult to justify CAM integration on economic grounds. Clearly one cannot separate perceptions of cost/benefit from views of effectiveness; but, given that the majority of these respondents used CAMs, it is reasonable to assume that they viewed them as potentially effective therapeutic options. Despite this, many did not see a role for them in the NHS. This tended to be because of the potential threat of further decline in the health service in terms of elective surgery or access to primary care. A significant proportion of those interviewed viewed CAMs (remembering, once again, that these are mostly CAM users) as a much lower priority than biomedical cancer care. This notion of the relative importance of CAM to its users is one that has tended to be underplayed. Recognition of this again confirms the importance of not assuming advocacy to be a logical corollary of use.

There is one further aspect to the data which adds a further dimension to the complexity about cost. When stage of disease was discussed, and particularly advanced disease, a much greater consistency in perspective was apparent:

PARTICIPANT: I think it just depends what stage of your disease you are at and on the individual patient because there will be patients in hospitals who would need someone like [name of spiritual healer] or some complementary therapy, they would need it in hospital, and then there are patients who have sort of moved on a step and are not requiring treatment at that time that, probably like the people that I have met, that didn't want to go back into the hospital environment and would prefer something like a complementary centre or something like that, out, you know, in the centre of [the city], you know, or out in the community.

(female, English, 57 years, breast)

An overwhelming majority of these patients viewed the provision of CAM to palliative care and advanced cancer patients (if indeed they desire such therapies) as fundamental. The economic cost/benefit was a significant issue in the context of patients with potentially curable disease but was considered absolutely irrelevant for patients with advanced disease. This is consistent with an interpretation of patient views which is based on their relative assessment of the appropriateness of expenditure. When cure is no longer considered possible, seemingly the tables are turned and the greater emotional, spiritual or just more rounded forms of CAM are established as the modalities of choice. Cost, given the relative perceived importance of CAM, therefore diminishes, if not disappears, as an issue.

Legitimacy of provider

Given that sporadic integration of CAM is already occurring in the UK, and that our sample included a substantial number of CAM users, we examined what respondents felt about that provision. We were specifically interested in views on where CAM was provided and by whom. All of the patients who participated in this study had access, via patient support centres, to selected CAMs. (Note that such services are highly limited and rationed according to prognosis and need.) However, in saying this, the majority were also using CAMs privately as well. Thus, they were in quite a unique position to provide feedback on the benefits of certain methods of delivery and how such processes could potentially be improved:

INTERVIEWER: For you, how would [CAM] best be delivered, in hospital or in the community?

PARTICIPANT: I think the thing about in-hospital is if you are going to hospital, it's fine, which is what I found with [the spiritual healer] when I was having the radiotherapy. Because I could do both at the same time. Once I wasn't going to that particular hospital, then the distance in travelling and the stress in travelling . . . you would get very stressed on a 20-mile journey there, de-stress and then get stressed up again on the way back home, so it kind of negated the benefits. But if it's delivered in the community I think that works well. The [cancer support centre] works well because it is not actually attached to the hospital so you go in and you don't feel like it's a hospital environment. You know, there aren't drips; there aren't nurses and doctors so it's more relaxed from that point of view. It's an escape from medicine but because it is near the hospital and because it is semi-official you trust the people who work there and you are prepared to travel to it . . . I mean, if you lived in the middle of nowhere, people aren't going to come to you, it would be too expensive. You have to accept that you are going to travel particularly if you are going to get it free. I think that is good because all the services are integrated so you are not having to go to a different place for each different thing. You can go for aromatherapy and while you are there somebody can say, 'Do you know you can claim benefits?', so you can do that, or you could go for an art class, and when you are finished your art class, then go for a reflexology session. So it becomes an alternative centre where you can do all the different things, meet different people, talk to different people.

(female, English, 51 years, bowel)

Another respondent:

PARTICIPANT: To me it's [hospital-located complementary medicine centre] quite a travel anyway. Well, it isn't too far, I mean, I do go. I was going kind of every day for a week at one stage. But I think actually it's good that it's with the hospital, to me. I think that's an advantage because you can just go round the corner and you are not leaving the hospital, especially where your wig and everything is concerned, I think it is also easier.

(female, English, 57 years, multiple myloma)

Another respondent:

PARTICIPANT: I think it [a complementary medicine service] would have to be something that was run by the NHS *and* out in the community, a health centre or a cancer centre community, BACUP centre or whatever they call them, you know the BACUP cancer care centres or something like that.

(female, English, 57 years, breast)

The complexity of responses is again in evidence here. For in a manner that would appear to be more supportive of the integration of CAM into state provision (than seen above), on the whole respondents tended to regard CAM therapists and the therapies they offer *within* NHS facilities to be safer and more trustworthy than those not affiliated to a Trust. Some patients recounted accepting the therapeutic potential of the CAMs offered without question, due to being offered them 'on site'. However, it should be remembered that respondents were being asked about existing integrative practice and the strengths and weaknesses of that, and not whether they believed CAMs should be sanctioned. As has already been shown, issues of evidence and cost make that much less clear cut.

Moreover, while the authority of provision under the NHS umbrella was widely highlighted, there was much less enthusiasm for such services to be spatially integrated with their biomedical treatment. As illustrated in the above excerpts, when asked where they would prefer CAMs to be delivered, many, although not all, respondents desired sites that were not on hospital grounds. Often they associated the hospital with their condition and viewed the CAM process as moving beyond their 'clinical diagnosis'. Moreover, on a practical level, for patients receiving debilitating chemotherapy, for example, travelling 20 miles to receive a relaxation therapy and then driving home was considered rather counterproductive. A common suggestion was that there should be NHS-sanctioned, community-based CAM therapists so that patients who live far away from the hospital site can get regular CAM therapies.

When turning to the legitimacy of various providers a further interesting point of differentiation emerged. On the one hand, patients interested in relaxation and healing therapies were generally highly supportive of CAM-trained nurses or NHS-sponsored CAM practitioners. However, on the other hand, those pursuing the more 'invasive' or 'rigorous' CAM regimes – viewed as more controversial than, say, the 'healing' therapies – often desired a complete separation between their biomedical care and CAM use (often due to perceptions of animosity between CAM and biomedicine):

INTERVIEWER: What do you think about the idea of nurses providing complementary therapies?

PARTICIPANT: Yes, if they're trained, yes. If they're trained; if they want to, yes.

INTERVIEWER: Would that be better, having nurses doing it in hospital, than, say, lay practitioners?

PARTICIPANT: Oh, I think the [complementary] practitioners have a place.

INTERVIEWER: What would make a lay practitioner different from a nurse practitioner?

PARTICIPANT: The person, isn't it, the person, yes. I mean, a nurse will have other duties and other demands. I mean, a lay practitioner would be focused on therapy, won't they, but I think the personality of the person makes a big difference . . . from my experience of going through complementary. . . . I think some people have a gift.

INTERVIEWER: Not just a skill but a gift?

PARTICIPANT: Yes, I think some people have a gift. They might be medical and they might not, it's the gift that matters.

(female, Scottish, 70 years, ovarian)

In relation to this latter group of respondents, a key theme that emerged from the interviews was that CAM could not necessarily be taught or learnt in a short course (and, in some cases, at all). The notion of the legitimacy of provision underpinned by the 'gift' held by certain CAM therapists was evident in many of these patients' accounts. The idea of CAM being taught to nurses or other allied health provisions was viewed as potentially meaning that it would lack a degree of authenticity. Moreover, as is shown in the above excerpt, there was a desire to separate the CAM world from that of the clinic, and the melding of biomedicine and CAM (say, using nursing staff) was viewed as potentially risking subsuming CAM within biomedical interventions. This desire to retain a sense of 'the other' in non-biomedical modalities for these respondents further undermines a simplistic notion of patient advocacy of CAM integration into state-funded cancer services *per se*.

Discussion

The aim of this chapter was to examine, empirically, the implicit assumption of cancer patients' support for the integration of CAM services into the NHS in the UK – an assumption influenced by a tendency to conflate use and advocacy. On the basis of this study we would argue that it is an oversimplification and indeed a distortion to present patient views in this way. While support for CAM as a set of therapeutic practices may well be strong, unequivocal support for integration into state-funded services does not inevitably follow from that. Assessment of the appropriateness of integration is instead mediated by engagement with the issues of evidence, risk, cost, location of provision and professional and epistemological identity of providers. Of course, this is a study firmly located in the UK context. While the headline issues discussed may well be relevant to CAM integration in other countries, empirical work within those countries is needed to test the relevance of our findings about those issues. The varying nature of mainstream provision to which integration relates (e.g. the level of state provision) in different countries may well impact on patient views (on, for instance, cost and the *relative* merits of CAM). We should also note that while our sample was large, it was limited to one region of the UK.

As use of CAM has increased exponentially over the last two decades despite the lack of evidence, it would seem reasonable to extrapolate from that that patients are satisfied to base personal decision-making on experiential knowledge rather than scientific evidence. And this study supports that. However, the finding that this does not automatically extend to patient views on the necessary basis for the integration of CAM therapies into state provision establishes an immediate need to reassess implicit or explicit assumptions that beliefs and actions at a personal level translate into beliefs about policy development. Moreover, it was not simply that evidence was seen as necessary to underpin integration. Instead, the picture was much more complex than that and bound up with perceptions of risk. Put simply, those approaches deemed to have more potential for harm were set higher standards (of support from controlled trials) than those deemed to be less risky.

Our next theme continued to demonstrate this complexity. The issue of economic cost created something of a split in terms of the perspectives of these patients, with a significant proportion viewing CAM integration as neither economically viable nor essential. This was particularly interesting given the fact that these were largely existing users of CAM. When faced with increased pressure on the NHS, many patients (and even CAM users) felt they could not support the increased costs incurred by CAM integration. The sense of the *relative* importance of CAM was pivotal here, as shown by the strength of support for the state provision of CAM at the end of life – when biomedicine no longer provided a meaningful option.

And finally, discussion of provider location and identity continued to demonstrate diversity and contingency of response. While a significant proportion of respondents were in favour of an NHS-regulated community-based form of CAM provision that would avoid the 'clinical feeling', there was also widespread acceptance that provision within the NHS offered a sense of security and regulation. Having said that, once beyond the more 'straightforward' therapies, many respondents held to the view that provision was best offered outside the system – not least because of the greater authenticity which such therapists were seen as having; an authenticity grounded in a practitioner's 'gift' as often as training, and one which might be undermined by subservience to biomedicine. Here again, the value of integration is frequently tempered by a sense that the benefits are not without cost.

These findings have important implications for policy development on the integration of CAM into state-funded cancer services. The inclusion of 'user perspectives' has become an integral part of policy rhetoric; it is important to acknowledge the complexity of such perspectives on the issue discussed in this chapter. Respondents in this study clearly operated with different approaches to the assessment of CAM at a personal level as opposed to a strategic level. Use cannot be taken as a simple proxy for advocacy. While patients may well have an appreciation of the intrinsic benefits of the approaches available, judgements about their integration are frequently grounded in real-world concerns such as limited resources, the need to fund the 'most important' modality at specific illness stages and so on. In short, when reaching beyond the surface of 'patient perspectives', a highly contingent, variable and complex picture emerges – one which should not be glossed over in the current integration-consensus driven environment.

7   Conclusion

Our aim in writing this book was to provide a sociologically informed analysis of the role CAMs are playing in cancer care in the UK. This was achieved by marrying a range of data sources to a critical engagement with various forms of sociological theory that have been drawn on when considering the place of CAMs in the West. We were able to draw on a substantial number of interviews with cancer patients and key oncology clinicians. Furthermore, we gathered in-depth diary data from a select group of these patients as a means of gaining insight into the day-to-day, temporal experiences of being a cancer patient, further expanding on our analysis of the face-to-face interviews. That the work is essentially sociological in nature is of some importance and represents a continuation of an approach to the study of CAM which has been detailed elsewhere (Tovey *et al.*, 2007). That approach is underpinned by the necessity of providing a form of analysis about CAMs that is focused neither on the pursuit of evidence on efficacy and effectiveness nor on the demands of immediate and localised policy agendas.

The book was structured so as to begin with chapters considering aspects of patient decision-making, to move on to analyses which brought forward the role of practitioners and then to consider the dynamic nature of processes before rounding off with an analysis of the complexity of integration. The opening empirical chapter has, at its core, what has perhaps become the central issue in debates about the future of CAM within mainstream healthcare provision – 'evidence'; specifically, in this case, the way in which cancer patients themselves engage with, and conceptualise, the issue and utilise different forms of evidence in relation to CAM and biomedicine. Central to our discussion has been an appreciation of the complexity inherent in cancer patients' ontological and epistemological positionings – positions that are influenced by the specifics of disease and treatment trajectories. While, for instance, there was much scepticism about an overreliance on statistical probabilities, this did not tend to constitute a fundamental rejection of their validity; rather, there was a critical awareness that what they meant for the patient as an individual was highly contingent. There was an emphasis on the subjective (and the need for hope) and a feeling that CAMs were frequently able to enter that space.

In the chapter which followed, we approached the issue of patient decision-making about CAM from a different angle. We examined the way in which the Internet is being used by patients to access information about CAM and biomedical cancer care. Surprisingly, up to this point no research had been conducted on this issue. This is especially surprising for us given that much of the rhetoric surrounding the use of the Internet has assumed its significant influence over patients (and cancer patients in particular) and the serious potential for patients to be exploited. Our results provided a rather different emphasis. Indeed, what emerged from this study was that previous assumptions that the Internet is a significant point of access to CAMs – bringing with it specific difficulties – is at best oversimplistic. In fact, for the patients in our sample access to biomedical knowledge frequently raised rather more problematic issues, particularly for users of CAM. Our results also had important implications for sociological theory and Internet studies more broadly. In particular, the data presented here throws serious doubt on the veracity of the claims of those social commentators who stress the role of the Internet in promoting therapeutic pluralism and thus contributing to the deprofessionalisation of medicine (or even reductions in biomedical power). In fact, the data presented here suggests the potential of the Internet as a virtual form of biomedicalisation, reinforcing the dominance of biomedical conceptions of disease.

Next, we shifted the focus on to cancer clinicians and began to consider how CAM integration is being operationalised in both the hospital and the hospice setting. Again, the use of 'evidence' proved to be central to the discussion and, in particular, to the ways in which differently positioned practitioners engage with, conceptualise and deploy 'evidence' in grassroots clinical settings. We demonstrated that the way in which the biomedical hierarchy of evidence is drawn on varies both between clinicians and, crucially, between types of organisation. In fact, we were able to illustrate how the structural characteristics of specific medical specialties (i.e. medical oncology versus palliative care) influence the utilisation of specific forms of evidence. In the hospital setting, for example, we saw the discursive deployment of 'evidence' and 'evidence-based medicine' as part of a process of professional gatekeeping. Evidence was used to underpin a strategy of differentiation and distinction between CAM and biomedicine. In the hospice, however, clinicians were far more willing to embrace patients' subjective needs, albeit within a framework of tight regulation for those practices enlisted. Importantly, therefore, the complexity which we'd already shown in patient action was being reflected in professional attitudes and behaviours – with strategic adaptation frequently evident.

As the next stage of our focus on clinicians we turned to how patients experienced interactions with doctors and nurses and the perceived impact of patient/clinician interactions on their engagement with CAM. Interestingly, not only did we find three broad types of response reported by patients – explicit or implicit negativity, supportive ambivalence and pragmatic acceptance – but we also discovered that patient accounts highlighted a clear influence on patient action from each of these. Our argument is not that patients automatically follow the diktat of oncologists, but instead that clinicians continue to play an important role in decision-making despite the theoretical possibility of influence from a range of other sources of information and from others making claims of expertise (i.e. CAM therapists). Indeed, the active engagement of cancer patients was shown clearly by the way in which alignment with specialist cancer nurses was developed as a counterweight to dynamics with oncologists in particular circumstances.

Until this point our analysis had been based on interview data. While valuable, such data does have the limitation of presenting only a snapshot of experience – the view of that individual respondent on the specific day in question. With this in mind, we rounded out our analysis through the collection of diary data from a small number of respondents. What this was able to provide was a sense of process – a reflection of the changing nature of patients' involvement with CAM. Indeed, the data revealed that experiences and perceptions of CAM are considerably more problematic than is sometimes revealed by more 'static' methods. The everyday act of 'doing CAM' is nuanced and complex. The adoption of this approach allowed us to discuss a number of issues that had hitherto remained undiscussed in the sociological literature, including potential disciplinary and self-governance processes within CAM therapeutics. The potential for the development of methods which reflect the dynamic nature of experience is clearly considerable.

In the final empirical chapter we considered directly the topic that is at the heart of much policy-level discussion of CAM and cancer care in the UK – the appropriateness of integration into mainstream healthcare provision. In particular we sought to critically explore the assumption that identifying significant levels of CAM use can be seen as providing supportive evidence that there is widespread patient enthusiasm for integration of CAM into the NHS. In so doing we were able to show that a characterisation of unequivocal support for integration amongst cancer patients (even amongst CAM users) is an oversimplification and distortion of the situation, and that 'use' and 'advocacy' need to remain conceptually distinct. By focusing on the building blocks of integration – evidence, risk, cost and provider legitimacy – patient engagement with the idea of integration was shown to be multi-layered. The implications for the current integration consensus were considered.

While each of these chapters had their own specific foci, a number of cross-cutting themes can be identified which are pivotal to an understanding of patient engagement with CAM, biomedicine and the clinicians responsible for the provision of care. First, in several chapters we have seen evidence of the continuing power of orthodox clinicians – and specifically of those in medicine. While much has been heard (both anecdotally and within theoretical discussions) of the plurality of experts, the threat to the power, authority and legitimacy of biomedical practitioners and the competing sources of information that patients can draw on, repeatedly in our study the continuing centrality of biomedical practitioners was apparent; evolving and adapting certainly, but still at the centre of patient action.

Second, despite this continuing influence of clinicians, agency and complexity in patient interaction with therapeutic options were seen time and again – particularly in relation to the flexible consideration of 'scientific' evidence, multidimensional assessments of integration and so on. While it may be of value to policymakers to try and pin down 'the' user perspective, such oversimplification clearly bears little resemblance to the variation and contingency found at grassroots level.

Third is the issue of integration. In addition to the chapter specifically assigned to the discussion of patient engagement with this concept, we saw how the structural characteristics of organisations (i.e. the hospital and the hospice) influenced the way in which CAM practices are incorporated and excluded on a day-to-day basis. In both cases the difficulties which can be anticipated for any policy which fails to take full account of individual and organisational dynamics were apparent.

And, fourth, in many areas of our analysis, issues relating to the conceptualisation, interpretation and utilisation of evidence were of major importance. Variously positioned participants demonstrated through their accounts how evidence is mediated in real-life contexts. The same 'piece' of evidence will have differing authority depending on a range of variables, including its application to policy-level or personal-level decision-making, the institutional context of its deployment and so on. Inherent in all the discussions were the limitations of a decontextualised understanding of how evidence may be used in relation to CAM and cancer.

The future agenda

Clearly there remains a substantial research agenda in the social or sociological analysis of the use of non-biomedical therapeutics by people with cancer. Indeed, our study discussed in this book has highlighted approaches and themes which might well be integral to this. For instance, while the majority of research in this (as in other areas) continues to provide a snapshot of experience, we have seen here the potential of approaches (in this case the diary method) to track changes and developments in the experience and actions of individuals. Such an approach can be usefully developed to help move further away from simplistic dualisms such as user/non-user to provide an insight into the ebb and flow which characterises engagement with CAM.

Beyond method, we can return to the cross-cutting themes outlined above to see areas in which much work is to be done. It was demonstrated, for example, how biomedical clinicians continue to play a powerful role in the decision-making processes of patients. Despite the increasing range of technological and professional sources of information and influence, we have seen how biomedical professionals continue to be central to decision-making. However, we need to understand in more detail the actual mechanisms through which this occurs and the extent to which variation within professions – on the basis of, for instance, disease specialism – is evident.

While the individual CAM user has been central to much of the existing work in this area, it is evident that a point has been reached in the research agenda when the agency and complexity at the heart of action need to be explored more fully. In interactions with clinicians, for example, alongside the influence of the professionals we saw an active mediation of events and information and at times selective alignments with certain biomedical practitioners.

With integration likely to remain a high-profile issue, we need to build on our findings, which illustrate complexity in patient perspectives, to examine further the priorities of patients. While we have explored dimensions on which patients make judgements about the appropriateness of integration into state-funded provision, many questions remain unanswered – not least about the impact that varying forms of inequality have on decision-making (a theme discussed more broadly in the next section).

And, of course, the issue of evidence also remains one in which further work is needed – especially in relation to policy initiatives on integration. While we have begun to unravel an approach to evidence assessment amongst patients which is multifaceted, this has yet to be taken further to an examination of what such patient perspectives suggest about the shape of the current CAM research agenda itself.

Over and above these issues, one theme in particular emerged from the present study as requiring more detailed attention – that of inequalities in relation to CAM consumption. We did not systematically approach the topic in our research and so our data is limited and should be treated as provisional and of value in suggesting questions for further research only. For this reason it is presented here rather than as a core part of our analysis.

Three biographical factors emerged from the perspectives of the patients interviewed as potentially influential in shaping perceptions of and access to CAM. These were socioeconomic status, gender and geographical location. Each of these factors, as explored in detail below, was seen as a mediating factor in both access to and experiences of CAM services (whether public or private).

Socioeconomic disadvantage and non-biomedical therapeutics

The first area that will require more detailed research is the relationship between socioeconomic status and CAM use. Perhaps unsurprisingly, given the basis of CAM provision in the private sector, what emerged from our patients' accounts was that CAM use was shaped by income and that, in large part, poorer patients and their carers missed out:

PARTICIPANT: The thing is I can't work any more, my husband's working, well, we go on caravan holidays because it is cheaper, we don't go abroad not any more . . . take going to [CAM therapist], I mean, I go every three weeks, which every three weeks isn't so bad paying every three weeks, but when I was going to go to acupuncture I was going to have to go three or four times a week. Well, that I just could not afford. I mean I get incapacity benefit but . . . I have still to pay for all my prescriptions . . . there's no way for me to keep that going.

(female, English, 55 years, melanoma)

Another respondent:

PARTICIPANT: I came out [of reflexology] feeling good . . . it made you feel . . . forget all about it and that, you know, it was good, it was wellbeing, it was nice.

INTERVIEWER: What stops you from getting that now?

PARTICIPANT: It's expensive and I don't want to pay out for having two things. I would rather go for my swim . . . You know, you have x amount of money and you are going to do A or B or C, and you might want to do something else, so therefore you stop doing that to do the other thing, you know, it's as simple as that . . . I would go every week . . . if there wasn't the cost.

(female, Irish, 69 years, bladder)

Although some participants found certain CAM therapies to be highly effective, it was financially difficult to access them. In cases of advanced disease, some, like those shown above, were on sickness benefits which allowed little room for expenses other than the most basic day-to-day necessities. In the case of the participants shown above, both of these cancer types (i.e. malignant melanoma and bladder cancer) have incredibly poor prognoses. However, participants had little or no ongoing access to complementary therapies due to cost. Both had initially been introduced to CAM through volunteer organisations offering limited sessions for free but then could not afford to support CAM use themselves. For these patients, and for a significant number of the other patients interviewed, this meant they had to decide between existing (albeit limited) leisure activities and CAM, the former usually taking precedence.

Self-funding and socioeconomic status

For those patients who had financial means, self-funding was often viewed as the only solution in a context of a paucity of NHS-provided services. Participants regularly reported spending thousands of pounds (for some, on a regular basis) in an attempt to 'get well' and 'fight their cancer'. In both the following excerpts we see patients with very advanced, 'incurable' disease talk about the financial impact of their use of CAMs:

PARTICIPANT: When I came back from Bristol [CAM clinic] they sent me a supplement pack and their basic supplement pack was £90 for a month, so you are putting a lot of money out. I mean this reverse osmosis filter is another £300 or £400. You can spend a lot of money and perhaps not get anywhere. But if you have got the money it feels like it is worth having a crack at it. You can always stop, can't you, and when I go shopping now, whilst I am buying organic things and it is costing me twice as much as ordinary, I am not buying the processed food.

INTERVIEWER: Do you think these therapies should be funded by the NHS?

PARTICIPANT: I do because, I mean, I can take advantage of it because I am in a privileged position but I think everybody should be able to if they want to, simple as that.

(female, English, 51 years, bowel)

Another respondent:

PARTICIPANT: Twice a week I have vitamin infusions, vitamins and minerals.

INTERVIEWER: How much would it cost you per month to do everything you are doing?

PARTICIPANT: So far it's cost us over £2,000.

INTERVIEWER: And you have been doing it for how long?

PARTICIPANT: Just over a month . . .

INTERVIEWER: How do you feel about that, having to pay for it?

PARTICIPANT: I don't mind it that much, although I would like the NHS to give us some money towards it because we are saving them thousands and thousands by not opting for medical treatments.

(male, English, 25 years, LP nodular Hodgkin's)

A significant proportion of the patients interviewed spent large amounts of money on CAM interventions, with many employing 'whole-system CAMs', which involve complete diet changes and special food processes and supplements. It was clear that although they did not *expect* the NHS to fund these treatment programmes they did view it as important to provide certain CAMs (i.e. the more inexpensive 'healing' CAMs) to patients who could not afford to pay themselves. An awareness of the privilege of certain wealthier patients was typical amongst the interviewers in the higher socioeconomic brackets. A system whereby patients pay a proportion of the cost, making CAM more accessible but still ensuring that patients contribute something (thereby minimising the potential for abuse of the system), was regularly suggested as a solution:

PARTICIPANT: Well, you see, I feel a little bit, I mean, we haven't got a lot of money, we have got a nice home and my husband is retired now . . . I would be quite willing to pay something towards anything like that [CAM therapies]. I mean if somebody said every time I went for reflexology, 'You will pay half of the cost', £5 or whatever, then I would do it. I mean, I personally would. To me it's worth the feeling that I got.

(female, English, 57 years, multiple myloma)

There was an overwhelming feeling amongst the interviewees that cancer patients would not take advantage of the system and, second, that most would be more than happy to contribute to the cost.

Ultimately, these patients perceived there to be 'haves' and 'have-nots' in relation to CAM; a system whereby private usage is significant amongst cancer patients but only amongst the wealthier groups. Although a 'free for all' system was not advocated by these patients, the necessity for a reassessment of the CAM needs of more disadvantaged groups was a clear theme.

The role of gender in mediating usage of and perceptions of CAM

There has been considerable speculation and some research on the role of gender in mediating attitudes towards, and the use of, CAM. However, as suggested earlier, most of this research has been disease specific (i.e. examining use and perceptions of female breast cancer patients) rather than examining patterns in perceptions amongst patients with a range of different conditions (e.g. Rees *et al.*, 2000). Moreover, previous studies have focused on the links between factors (i.e. gender and CAM use) rather than the actual processes underpinning these very links.

Our provisional data suggests that both engagement with and experiences of CAM may be mediated by gender constructs. Both the men and the women interviewed here discussed the gendered nature of CAM engagement, the tendency of men to resist certain features of CAM and the relationship of this resistance to idealised (and potentially hegemonic) constructions of masculinity:

PARTICIPANT: I think a woman is more open to take it [CAM] than a man really.

INTERVIEWER: Why do you think that is?

PARTICIPANT: It's probably a macho thing, isn't it? You know, I don't need them sort of things, they are women's things. Oh, I feel like my wife is a lot harder than I am. They can stand more can't they, they are . . .

INTERVIEWER: What do you think would make them women's things? I mean, versus . . . you know, what makes them more sort of orientated around women than men . . . therapies like aromatherapy or healing therapies or reiki or whatever?

PARTICIPANT: Aromatherapy, well, to be quite honest I don't really know exactly what aromatherapy is. When my wife talks about aromatherapy – she doesn't go to it by the way – and the first thing that came into my mind was having being rubbed down by scented oils.

INTERVIEWER: It's basically what it is.

PARTICIPANT: Well, why would men want to do that?

INTERVIEWER: It's not something that men would sort of traditionally have done to them really, is it?

PARTICIPANT: No, not really, that's why I say it is more of a woman thing, isn't it? [laughs]. . . . I mean, I can see you being rubbed down with anything that has not got perfume in it, don't get me wrong, I mean, they do it to footballers and rugby players and boxers, don't they, with camphorated oil and all that sort of thing, you know? But I can't see perfumed oils being right good.

(male, English, 68 years, prostate)

Another respondent:

PARTICIPANT: Men don't believe a lot in spirit and body and mind healing . . . I think if they are really, really desperate, if they are really maybe dying or terminal they would think about considering it, but they are always very apprehensive about . . . I think women sort of care more about their bodies, I suppose, than men. Men just think it's for football, kicking, sex or other thing. Well, forget about caring inside your body.

(female, Serbian, 51 years, breast)

Another respondent:

PARTICIPANT: Yes, I think, I think women are constantly striving through, whether they like to think it or not, they are constantly striving for an enhanced state mainly because of peer pressure, media pressure . . . you hear your friends and other people talking about [complementary medicine], you read about it in magazines, you think, maybe I'll try it . . . I don't think that men think about things at that level and from what I see a lot of men that do follow, say, the aromatherapy or the reflexology route are there because they have been encouraged to by their wives or their partners.

(female, English, 61 years, ovarian)

There was a clear sense in the interviews that gender was influential in mediating attitudes towards CAM – this was evident in the accounts of both the men and the women interviewed. The key facets of CAM that were described as particularly problematic for dominant constructions of masculinity were 'spirituality', 'touch' and 'perfumed oils'. These were characterised as counter to prevailing constructions of manliness and ultimately led to men rejecting CAM interventions.

On another level, the CAM field was perceived as being merely another reflection of the tendency of men not to access support and acknowledge illness. Thus, rather than being a 'special case', the tendency of men to 'shy away' from CAM use or perceive it as 'rather girly' was merely a reflection of wider patterns in health behaviour. The nature of CAM was not the issue *per se*, but rather wider differentiation in access to health services.

A third and important theme was the notion of women identifying more with anecdote and focusing less on scientific evidence:

PARTICIPANT: Probably, I mean, I don't think I'm that conscious of it, but I can understand why men don't use complementary therapies as much, because men tend not to, you know ... I don't know, I suppose for me what's important is not just the scientific but also intuitive. You know, there's lots of things that are happening in your body that we don't understand like the mind–body interaction, you know, so I'm prepared to, you know, take that leap of faith and whether that's a female thing or not I don't know. But there's also, certainly, in the women's magazines and with women that you talk to there's a lot of discussion about, you know, whether it's diet and keeping off dairy foods or, you know, using some of these complementary therapies or whatever. So I suppose in that sense there's a link.

(female, English, 50 years, breast)

The men expressed a degree of scepticism and/or awkwardness in relation to touch, healing or massage therapies, although for those who had advanced disease this seemed to dissipate.

Geographical location and equity in access to CAM services

As suggested previously, the 'postcode lottery' or differentiation according to geographical location in the UK has been a key issue in healthcare planning and political debate over the last decade in particular. It has long been recognised that patients who live in the 'catchment zones' for major teaching hospitals tend to receive more effective treatment and social support services. As with cancer care in general, from the perspectives of these patients the issue of geographical location was raised as relevant to accessing CAMs. A major source of CAMs (particularly for the lower socioeconomic groups) is volunteer-organisation-funded support centres in teaching hospitals. Clearly, these services are restricted, and for some patients are largely inaccessible due to travel. The effort to get to the sessions provided, according to some patients, made the effect of the therapy largely insignificant:

PARTICIPANT: Once I wasn't going to that particular hospital, then the distance in travelling and the stress in travelling, you would get very stressed up on a 20-mile journey there, de-stress and then get stressed up again on the way back home, so it kind of negated the benefits.

(female, English, 51 years, bowel)

Given the centralisation of NHS-funded or subsided CAM services in the major teaching hospitals, patients in smaller cities and rural areas may have little or no access given the practicalities involved. The time taken to access social support services may actually create more stress and anxiety and negate the therapeutic benefits of the particular CAMs.

Clearly there is need to study these dimensions of inequalities and CAM in much more detail. While there is enough in our own data to highlight the potential significance of the issues of socioeconomic status, gender and geography, further and more specifically focused work is needed to tease out these issues and processes in more depth.

Finally, it is important to reiterate that most research attention remains on the generation of 'evidence' concerning effectiveness and efficacy rather than on the sociological processes which impinge on and shape the utilisation of that evidence. As a consequence, the sociological study of CAM and cancer remains underdeveloped and the above represents merely a part of the extensive future research agenda in this field.

Notes

3 Integrating CAM: a comparative analysis of hospice versus hospital medicine

1 Given the prominence of the randomised controlled trial, or RCT, in the accounts presented here, some clarification of what this catergory means in practice is useful at this point. 'Testing' an intervention by comparing a treatment group (which receives an intervention) with a control group (which receives no treatment or a placebo), and possibly using a third group that receives standard care, is *generally* viewed within the biomedical community as producing the most 'scientifically' valid evidence of effectiveness. Where participants are allocated to these groups randomly, the experiment is a randomised controlled trial. An RCT may be single/double/ triple/quadruple blind depending on how many groups (i.e. patients, caregivers or assessors) are 'blinded', i.e. the information regarding the distribution/allocation of treatments involved in the RCT is kept from them. RCTs are of either a parallel, cross-over or factorial design. A parallel RCT involves testing the particular intervention in parallel with a placebo/control. A cross-over design involves all participants receiving each of the interventions in successive periods. Cross-over trials produce within-participant comparisons, whereas parallel designs produce between-participant comparisons. An RCT has a factorial design when two or more interventions are being tested, in combination, against each other and against a placebo/control.

5 Exploring the temporal dimension in cancer patients' experiences of non-biomedical therapeutics

1 The Gerson diet is a diet devised by Max Gerson and is very controversial amongst the mainstream biomedical community. Gerson believed that cancer and other degenerative and autoimmune diseases are caused by chronic malfunctions in cell metabolism, and that they can be effectively treated by restoring proper cell functioning through a diet which is high in potassium and low in sodium. He advised a diet of fresh vegetables and fruit, with minimum cooking and ideally without animal or dairy products, fats or sugars. The costs of the diet are considerable (particularly for treatment in a 'Gerson clinic') and treatment can have serious side-effects, including infections, dehydration and fitting. There is currently no scientific evidence to back up its efficacy in treating any form of cancer. The following is what the Gerson diet asks patients to consume daily: 2×200 cc fresh calf's liver juice; 4×200 cc green leaf juice; 5×200 cc apple and carrot juice; 1×200 cc orange or grapefruit juice. Forbidden items include tobacco, salt, tea, coffee, cocoa, chocolate, alcohol, white sugar, white flour, candy, ice cream, cream, cake, nuts, mushrooms, soybeans and soy products, cucumbers and pumpkins, pineapples, all

berries (except redcurrants). Furthermore, anything that is canned, bottled, sulphured, frozen, smoked, salted or bleached is banned. Patients are also not allowed to consume fat, oil, salt substitutes, bicarbonate of soda, or dye their hair. On top of these things, the following are temporarily forbidden during the first months of treatment: meat, fish, eggs, butter, cheese and milk. See Gerson, 1954.

Bibliography

Abbott, A. (1988) *The System of Professions: An Essay on the Division of Expert Labor*, Chicago: University of Chicago Press.

Adams, J. (ed.) (2007) *Researching Complementary and Alternative Medicine*, London and New York: Routledge.

Adams, J., Sibbritt, D., Easthope, G. and Young, A. (2003) 'The profile of women who consult alternative health practitioners in Australia', *Medical Journal of Australia*, 179(6): 297–300.

Adams, J., Sibbritt, D. and Young, A. (2005) 'Naturopathy/herbalism consultations by mid-age women who have cancer', *European Journal of Cancer Care*, 14: 443–7.

Addington-Hall, J. and Karlsen, S. (2005) 'A national survey of health professionals and volunteers working in voluntary hospice services in the UK', *Palliative Medicine*, 19(1): 40–8.

Adler, S. and Fosket, J. (1999) 'Disclosing complementary and alternative medicine use in the medical encounter: a qualitative study in women with breast cancer', *Journal of Family Practice*, 48: 453–8.

Agre, P. (2002) 'Real-time politics: the Internet and the political process', *The Information Society*, 18(5): 311–31.

Alferi, S., Antoni, M, Ironson, G., Kilbourn, K. and Carver, C. (2001) 'Factors predicting the use of complementary therapies in a multi-ethnic sample of early stage breast cancer patients', *Journal of the American Medical Women's Association*, 56: 120–3.

Anderson, J., Rainey, M. and Eysenbach, G. (2003) 'The impact of cyberhealthcare on the physician/patient relationship', *Journal of Medical Systems*, 27(1): 67–84.

Anspach, R. (1988) 'Notes on the sociology of medical discourse', *Journal of Health and Social Behaviour*, 29: 357–5.

Armstrong, N. (2007) 'Discourse and the individual in cervical cancer screening', *Health*, 11: 69–85.

Arora, N. (2003) 'Interacting with cancer patients: the significance of physicians' communication behaviour', *Social Science & Medicine*, 57: 791–806.

Astin, J., Marie, A., Pelletier, K., Hansen, E. and Haskell, W. (1998) 'A review of the incorporation of complementary and alternative medicine by mainstream physicians', *Archives of Internal Medicine*, 158(21): 2303–10.

Bain, K., Weschules, D., Knowlton, C. and Gallagher, R. (2003) 'Toward evidence-based prescribing at end of life', *American Journal of Hospice & Palliative Care*, 20(5): 382–8.

Baird, A., Donnelly, C., Miscampell, N. and Wemyss, H. (2000) 'Centralisation of cancer services in rural areas has disadvantages', *British Medical Journal*, 320: 717.

Bakx, K. (1991) 'The "eclipse" of folk medicine in western society', *Sociology of Health & Illness*, 13(1): 20–38.

Banning, M. (2005) 'Conceptions of evidence, evidence-based medicine, evidence-based practice and their use in nursing: independent nurse prescribers' views', *Journal of Clinical Nursing*, 7: 411–17.

Barnes, P.M., Powell-Griner, E., McFann, K. and Nahin, R.L. (2004) 'Complementary and alternative medicine use among adults: United States, 2002', *Advance Data*, May 27(343): 1–19.

Barry, A. (2006) 'The role of evidence in alternative medicine: contrasting biomedical and anthropological approaches', *Social Science & Medicine*, 62(11): 2646–57.

Basch, E., Thaler, H., Shi, W., Yakren, S. and Schrag, D. (2004) 'Use of information resources by patients with cancer and their companions', *Cancer*, 1000(11): 2476–83.

Baum, M. (2004) 'An open letter to the Prince of Wales: with respect, your highness, you've got it wrong', *British Medical Journal*, 329: 118.

Baum, M. (2006) 'Use of "alternative" medicine in the NHS', *The Times*, 23 May.

Beck, U. (1992) *Risk Society: Towards a New Modernity*, London: Sage.

Begley, C. (1996) 'Triangulation of communication skills in qualitative research instruments', *Journal of Advanced Nursing*, 24: 688–93.

Beider, S. (2005) 'An ethical argument for integrated palliative care', *Evidence Based Complementary and Alternative Medicine*, 2(2): 227–31.

Beisecker, A. and Beisecker, T. (1990) 'Patient information-seeking behaviours when communicating with doctors', *Medical Care*, 28: 19–28.

Berger, P. and Luckmann, T. (1967) *The Social Construction of Reality: A Treatise in the Sociology of Knowledge*, London: Allen Lane.

Berman, B. (2003) 'Integrative approaches to pain management: how to get the best of both worlds', *British Medical Journal*, 326: 1320–1.

Bernstein, B. and Grasso, T. (2001) 'Prevalence of complementary and alternative medicine use in cancer patients', *Oncology*, 15(10): 1272–83.

Bernstein, J. and Shuval, J. (1997) 'Non-conventional medicine in Israel: consultation patterns of the Israeli population and attitudes of primary care physicians', *Social Science & Medicine*, 44(9): 1341–8.

Bishop, F. and Yardley, L. (2004) 'Constructing agency in treatment decisions', *Health*, 8(4): 465–82.

Bombardieri, D. and Easthope, G. (2000) 'Convergence between orthodox and alternative medicine', *Health*, 4(4): 479–94.

Boon, H., Brown, J., Gavin, A., Kennard, M. and Stewart, M. (1999) 'Breast cancer survivors' perceptions of complementary/alternative medicine (CAM): making the decision to use or not to use', *Qualitative Health Research*, 9(5): 639–53.

Boon, H., Stewart, M., Kennard, M., Gray, R., Sawka, C., Brown, J., McWilliam, C., Gavin, A., Baron, R., Aaron, D. and Haines-Kamka, T. (2000) 'Use of complementary/alternative medicine by breast cancer survivors in Ontario: prevalence and perceptions', *Journal of Clinical Oncology*, 18(13): 2515–21.

Boon, H., Welsh, S., Kelner, M. and Wellman, B. (2004) 'Complementary and alternative practitioners and the professionalisation process', in Tovey, P., Easthope, G. and Adams, J. (eds) *The Mainstreaming of Complementary and Alternative Medicine*, London: Routledge.

Borgerson, K. (2005) 'Evidence-based alternative medicine?', *Perspectives in Biology and Medicine*, 48(4): 502–15.

Boschma, G. (1994) 'The meaning of holism in nursing: historical shifts in holistic nursing ideas', *Public Health Nursing*, 11(5): 324–30.

Bradlow, A., Coulter, A. and Brooks, P. (1992) *Patterns of Referral*, Oxford: Health Services Research Unit.

Broom, A. (2002) 'Contested territories: the construction of boundaries between "alternative" and "conventional" cancer treatments', *New Zealand Journal of Sociology*, 17: 215–34.

Broom, A. (2004) 'Prostate cancer and masculinity in Australian society: a case of stolen identity?', *International Journal of Men's Health*, 3(2): 73–91.

Broom, A. (2005) 'Medical specialists' accounts of the impact of the Internet on the doctor/patient relationship', *Health*, 9(3): 319–38.

Broom, A. (2005a) 'Virtually he@lthy: a study into the impact of Internet use on disease experience and the doctor/patient relationship', *Qualitative Health Research*, 15(3): 325–45.

Broom, A. (2005b) 'The eMale: prostate cancer, masculinity and online support as a challenge to medical expertise', *Journal of Sociology*, 41(1): 87–104.

Broom, A. (2005c) 'Using qualitative interviews in complementary and alternative medicine research: a guide to study design, data collection and data analysis', *Complementary Therapies in Medicine*, 13(1): 65–73.

Broom, A. (2006) 'Reflections on the centrality of power in medical sociology: an empirical test and theoretical elaboration', *Health Sociology Review*, 15(5): 55–70.

Broom, A. (2006a) 'The impact of the Internet on patients' expectations', *Nature Clinical Practice Urology*, 3(3): 117.

Broom, A. (2006b) 'Ethical issues in social research', *Complementary Therapies in Medicine*, 13(1): 151–6.

Broom, A. and Adams, J. (2007) 'Researching complementary medicine: current issues and future directions', *Complementary Therapies in Medicine*, 15(1): 1–7.

Broom, A. and Tovey, P. (2007) 'Therapeutic pluralism? Evidence, power and legitimacy in UK cancer services', *Sociology of Health & Illness*, 29(4): 551–69.

Broom, A. and Tovey, P. (2007a) 'The dialectical tension between individuation and depersonalisation in cancer patients' mediation of complementary, alternative and biomedical cancer treatments', *Sociology*, 41(6): 1–20.

Broom, A. and Tovey, P. (forthcoming) 'The role of the Internet in cancer patients' engagement with complementary and alternative treatments', *Health*.

Broom, A., Barnes, J. and Tovey, P. (2004) 'Introduction to research methods in CAM series', *Complementary Therapies in Medicine*, 12(2): 165–73.

Bryman, A. and Burgess, R. (1994) *Analysing Qualitative Data*, London: Routledge

Burgers, J., Fervers, B., Haugh, M., Brouwers, M., Browman, G., Philip, T. and Cluzeau, F. (2004) 'International assessment of the quality of clinical practice guidelines in oncology using the Appraisal of Guidelines and Research and Evaluation Instrument', *Journal of Clinical Oncology*, 22(10): 2000–7.

Burstein, H. (2000) 'Discussing complementary therapies with cancer patients: what should we be talking about?', *Journal of Clinical Oncology*, 18(13): 2501–4.

Burstein, H., Gelber, S., Guadagnoli, E. and Weeks, J. (1999) 'Use of alternative medicine by women with early stage breast cancer', *New England Journal of Medicine*, 340: 1733–9.

Burrows, R., Nettleton, S., Pleace, N., Pleace, N. and Muncer, S. (2000) 'Virtual community care: social policy and the emergence of computer mediated social support', *Information, Communication and Society*, 3(1): 95–121.

Cahoone, L. (1996) *From Modernism to Postmodernism: An Anthology*, Oxford: Blackwell Publishers.

Calnan, M., Montaner, D. and Horne, R. (2005) 'How acceptable are innovative health-care technologies? A survey of public beliefs and attitudes in England and Wales', *Social Science & Medicine*, 60: 1937–48.

Cameron, E. and Bernardes, J. (1998) 'Gender and disadvantage in health: men's health for a change', *Sociology of Health & Illness*, 20(5): 673–93.

Cancer Research Campaign (1999) *CancerStats: Survival England and Wales 1971–1995*, London: CRC.

Cant, S. and Calnan, M. (1991) 'On the margins of the medical marketplace? An exploratory study of alternative practitioners' perceptions', *Sociology of Health & Illness*, 13(1): 39–57.

Canter, P., Thompson-Coon, J. and Ernst, E. (2005) 'Cost effectiveness of complementary treatments in the United Kingdom: systematic review', *British Medical Journal*, 331: 880–1.

Carlile, S. and Sefton, A. (1998) 'Healthcare and the information age: implications for medical education', *Medical Journal of Australia*, 168: 340–3.

Carlson, L., Speca, M., Patel, K. and Goodey, E. (2004) 'Mindfulness-based stress reduction in relation to quality of life', *Psychoneuroendocrinology*, 29(4): 448–74.

Carlsson, M. (2000) 'Cancer patients seeking information from sources outside the healthcare system', *Support Care in Cancer*, 8: 453–7.

Cartwright T. (2007) '"Getting on with life": the experiences of older people using complementary healthcare', *Social Science & Medicine*, 64(8): 1692–703.

Caspi, O., Bell, I., Rychener, D., Gaudet, T. and Weil, A. (2000) 'The tower of Babel: communication and medicine: an essay on medical education and complementary/alternative medicine', *Archives of Internal Medicine*, 160: 3193–5.

Cassileth, B. and Deng, G. (2004) 'Complementary and alternative therapies for cancer', *The Oncologist*, 9(1): 80–9.

Cassileth, B. and Vickers, A (2005) 'High prevalence of complementary and alternative medicine use among cancer patients: implications for research and clinical care', *Journal of Clinical Oncology*, 23(12): 2590–2.

Charmaz, K. (1990) '"Discovering" chronic illness: using grounded theory', *Social Science & Medicine*, 30(11): 1161–72.

Chatwin, J. and Tovey, P. (2004) 'Complementary and alternative medicine (CAM), cancer and group-based action: a critical review of the literature', *European Journal of Cancer Care*, 13: 210–18.

Chen, X. and Siu, L. (2001) 'Impact of the media and the internet on oncology: survey of cancer patients and oncologists in Canada', *Journal of Clinical Oncology*, 19(23): 4291–7.

Cherlin, E., Fried, T., Prigerson, H., Schulman-Green, D., Johnson-Hurzeler, R. and Bradley, E. (2005) 'Communication between physicians and family caregivers about care at the end of life: when do discussions occur and what is said?', *Journal of Palliative Medicine*, 8(6): 1176–85.

Chiu, P. and Mok, E. (2004) 'Nurse–patient relationships in palliative care', *Journal of Advanced Nursing*, 48(5): 475–83.

Chong, O. (2006) 'An integrative approach to addressing clinical issues in complementary and alternative medicine in an outpatient oncology center', *Clinical Journal of Oncology Nursing*, 10(1): 83–8.

Clayton, A. and Thorne, T. (2000) 'Diary data enhancing rigour: analysis framework and verification tool', *Journal of Advanced Nursing*, 32(6): 1514–21.

Cline, R. and Haynes, K. (2001) 'Consumer health information seeking on the Internet: the state of the art', *Health Education Research*, 16(6): 671–92.

Cooke, B. and Ernst, E. (2000) 'Aromatherapy: a systematic review', *British Journal of General Practice*, June: 493–6.

Corner, J., Cawley, N. and Hildebrand, S. (1995) 'An evaluation of the use of massage and essential oils on the wellbeing of cancer patients', *International Journal of Palliative Nursing*, 1(2): 67–73.

Corti, L. (1993) 'Using diaries in social research', *Social Research Update*, 2; available online: http://www.soc.surrey.ac.uk/sru/sru2.html.

Cotton, S. (2001) 'Implications of Internet technology for medical sociology in the new millennium', *Sociological Spectrum*, 21: 319–40.

Coulter, I. (2004) 'Integration and paradigm clash', in Tovey, P., Easthope, G. and Adams, J. (eds), *The Mainstreaming of Complementary and Alternative Medicine*, London, Routledge.

Coulter, I. and Willis, E. (2004) 'The rise and rise of complementary and alternative medicine: a sociological perspective', *Medical Journal of Australia*, 180: 587–9.

Court, C. (1995) 'Survey reveals men's ignorance about health', *British Medical Journal*, 310: 759.

Cox, J. (2000) 'Evidence in oncology: the Janeway lecture', *Cancer Journal*, 6(6): 351–7.

Crock, R., Jarjoura, D., Polen, A. and Rutecki, G. (1999) 'Confronting the communication gap between conventional and alternative medicine: a survey of physicians' attitudes', *Alternative Therapies in Health and Medicine*, 5: 61–6.

CRUK (2006) *UK cancer incidence statistics*, Cancer Research UK; available online: http://info.cancerresearchuk.org/cancerstats/incidence/.

Davidson, R., Geoghegan, L., McLaughlin, L. and Woodward, R. (2005) 'Psychological characteristics of cancer patients who use complementary therapies', *Psycho-Oncology*, 14: 187–95.

Department of Health (2000) *NHS Cancer Plan*, London: Department of Health.

Department of Health (2004) *The NHS Cancer Plan and the New NHS*, London: Department of Health.

Dew, K. (1997) 'Limits on the utilization of alternative therapies by doctors: a problem of boundary maintenance', *Australian Journal of Social Issues* 32(2): 181–97.

Dew, K. (1998) *Borderland Practices: Validating and Regulating Alternative Therapies in New Zealand*, PhD thesis in Sociology, Wellington: Victoria University of Wellington.

Dew, K. (2000) 'Apostasy to orthodoxy: debates before a commission of inquiry into chiropractic', *Sociology of Health & Illness*, 22(3): 310–30.

Dew, K. (2000a) 'Deviant insiders: medical acupuncturists in New Zealand', *Social Science & Medicine*, 50(12): 1785–95.

Diaz, J., Griffith, R., Ng, J., Reinert, S., Friedmann, P. and Moulton, A. (2002) 'Patients' use of the Internet for medical information', *Journal of General Internal Medicine*, 17: 180–5.

Djulbegovic, B. and Sullivan, D. (eds) (1997) *Decision-Making in Oncology. Evidence-based Management*, New York: Churchill Livingstone.

Djulbegovic, B., Loughran, T. and Hornung C. *et al.* (1999) 'The quality of medical evidence in hematology-oncology', *American Journal of Medicine*, 106: 198–205.

Dobbie, A., Schneider, F., Anderson A.D. and Littlefield, J. (2000) 'What evidence supports teaching evidence-based medicine?', *Academic Medicine*, 75(12): 1184–5.

Doel, M. and Segrott, J. (2003) 'Self, health and gender: complementary and alternative medicine in the British mass media', *Gender, Place and Culture: A Journal of Feminist Geography*, 10(2): 131–44.

Dudley, T., Falvo, D., Podell, R. and Renner, J. (1996) 'The informed patient poses a different challenge', *Patient Care*, 30(19): 128–38.

Eastwood, H. (2000) 'Postmodernisation, consumerism and the shift towards holistic health', *Journal of Sociology*, 36: 133–55.

Elliott, H. (1997) 'The use of diary methods in sociological research on health experience', *Sociological Research Online*, 2(2); available online: http://www.socresonline.org.uk/socresonline/2/2/7.html (accessed 7 February 2007).

Eng, J., Ramsum, D., Verhoef, M., Guns, E., Davison, J. and Gallagher, R. (2003) 'A population-based survey of complementary and alternative medicine use in men recently diagnosed with prostate cancer', *Integrative Cancer Therapies*, 2(3): 212–16.

Ernst, E. (2000) 'The role of complementary and alternative medicine', *British Medical Journal*, 321: 1133–5.

Ernst, E. (2001) *The Desktop Guide to CAM*, Edinburgh: Mosby.

Ernst, E. (2001a) 'Complementary therapies in palliative cancer care', *Cancer*, 91(11): 2181–5.

Ernst, E. (2002) 'The risk–benefit profile of commonly used herbal therapies: ginkgo, St. John's wort, ginseng, echinacea, saw palmetto, and kava', *Annals of Internal Medicine*, 1136(1): 42–53.

Ernst, E. (2005) 'Is homeopathy a clinically valuable approach?', *Trends in Pharmacological Sciences*, 26(11): 547–8.

Ernst, E. (2005a) 'Second thoughts on integrative medicine', *Journal of Family Practice*, 54(2): 154–5.

Ernst, E., and Cassileth, S. (1998) 'The prevalence of complementary/alternative medicine in cancer: a systematic review', *Cancer*, 83: 777–82.

Ernst, E. and Schmidt, K. (2002) '"Alternative" cancer cures via the Internet?' *British Journal of Cancer*, 87: 479–80.

Eysenbach G. (2003) 'The impact of the Internet on cancer outcomes', *CA: A Cancer Journal for Clinicians*, 53(6): 356–71.

Ezzy, D. (2002) *Qualitative Analysis: Practice and Innovation*, St Leonards, NSW: Allen and Unwin.

Filshie, J. (1990) 'Acupuncture for malignant pain', *Acupuncture in Medicine*, 8(2): 38–9.

Foucault, M. (1988) 'Technologies of the self', in Martin, Luther H., Gutman, Huck and Hutton, Patrick H. (eds) *Technologies of the Self: A Seminar with Michel Foucault*, Amherst, MA: The University of Massachusetts Press.

Fouladbakhsh, J., Stommel, M., Given, B. and Given, C. (2005) 'Predictors of use of complementary and alternative therapies among patients with cancer', *Oncology Nursing Forum*, 32(6): 1115–22.

Foundation for Integrated Medicine (2006) *Integrated Healthcare: A Way Forward for the Next Five Years?*, London: Foundation for Integrated Medicine.

Fox, N. and Roberts, C. (1999) 'GPs in cyberspace: the sociology of the virtual community', *Sociological Review*, 47(4): 643–71.

Fox, N., Ward, K. and O'Rourke, A. (2005) 'The "expert patient": empowerment or medical dominance? The case of weight loss, pharmaceutical drugs and the Internet', *Social Science & Medicine*, 60: 1299–309.

Fox, S. (2005) *Health information online*, Washington, DC: Pew Internet and American Life Project.

Foy, R., So, J., Rous, E. and Scarffe, J. (1999) 'Perspectives of commissioners and cancer specialists in prioritising new cancer drugs', *British Medical Journal*, 318(7181): 456–9.

Frenkel, M. and Borkan, J. (2003) 'An approach for integrating complemetary–alternative medicine into primary care', *Family Practice*, 20: 324–32.

Frisch, N. (2001) 'Standards for holistic nursing practice: a way to think about our care that includes complementary and alternative modalities', *Online Journal of Issues in Nursing*, 6(2); available online: http://www.nursingworld.org/ojin/topic15/tpc15_4.htm.

FTC (2001) *Health Claims on the Internet: Buyer Beware*, Washington, DC: Federal Trade Commission.

Fulder, S. (1996) *The Handbook of Alternative and Complementary Medicine*, 3rd edn, Oxford: Oxford University Press.

Geertz, C. (1973) *The Interpretation of Cultures: Selected Essays*, New York: Basic Books.

Germov, J. (1995) 'Medifraud, managerialism and the decline of medical autonomy', *Australia and New Zealand Journal of Sociology*, 31(3): 51–66.

Gerson, M. (1954) 'Cancer, a problem of metabolism', *Medizinische Klinik*, 49(26): 1028–32.

Giddens, A. (1990) *The Consequences of Modernity*, Cambridge: Polity Press.

Giddens, A. (1991) *Modernity and Self-identity: Self and Society in the Late Modern Age*, Stanford: Stanford University Press.

Gilliam, A., Speake, W., Scholefield, J. and Beckingham, I. (2003) 'Finding the best from the rest: evaluation of the quality of patient information on the Internet', *Annals of the Royal College of Surgeons England*, 85: 44–6.

Girgis, A., Adams, J. and Sibbritt, D. (2005) 'The use of complementary and alternative therapies by patients with cancer', *Oncology Research*, 15(15): 281–9.

Glaser, B. and Strauss, (1967) *The Discovery of Grounded Theory: Strategies for Qualitative Research*, Chicago: Aldine Publishing Company.

Goldenberg, M. (2006) 'On evidence and evidence-based medicine', *Social Science and Medicine*, 62(11): 2621–32.

Goldstein, M. (2004) 'The persistence and resurgence of medical pluralism', *Journal of Health Politics, Policy and Law*, 29: 925–45.

Goldszmidt, M., Levitt, C., Duarte-Franco, E. and Kaczorowski, J. (1995) 'Complementary healthcare services: a survey of general practitioners' views', *Canadian Medical Association Journal*, 1153: 29–35.

Gray, D. (2002) 'Deprofessionalising doctors? The independence of the British medical profession is under unprecedented attack', *British Medical Journal*, 324(7338): 627–9.

Gubrium, J. and Holstein, J. (1997) *The New Language of Qualitative Method*, New York: Oxford University Press.

Hack, T., Degnera, L. and Parker, P. (2005) 'The communication goals and needs of cancer patients: a review', *Psycho-Oncology*, 14: 831–45.

Hall, E. (2005) 'The "geneticisation" of heart disease: a network analysis of the production of new genetic knowledge', *Social Science & Medicine*, 60: 2673–83.

Hampsten, E. (1989) 'Considering more than a single reader', in Personal Narratives Group (ed.), *Interpreting Women's Lives: Feminist Theory and Personal Narratives*, Bloomington: Indiana University Press.

Hann, D., Baker, F. and Denniston, M. (2003) 'Oncology professionals' communication with cancer patients about complementary therapy: a survey', *Complementary Therapies in Medicine*, 11: 184–90.

Hardey, M. (1999) 'Doctor in the house: the Internet as a source of health knowledge and a challenge to expertise', *Sociology of Health & Illness*, 21(6): 820–35.

Hardey, M. (2002) ' "The story of my illness": personal accounts of illness on the Internet', *Health*, 6(1): 31–46.

Hardy, M., Coulter, I., Venuturupalli, S., Roth, E., Favreau, J., Morton, S. and Shekelle, P. (2001) *Ayurvedic Interventions for Diabetes Mellitus: A Systematic Review*, Santa Monica, CA: Southern California Evidence-Based Practice Center, RAND.

Harris, P., Finlay, I., Cook, A., Thomas, K. and Hood, K. (2003) 'Complementary and alternative medicine use by patients with cancer in Wales: a cross sectional survey', *Complementary Therapies in Medicine*, 11(4): 249–53.

Harrison, J., Maguire, P. and Pitceathly, C. (1995) 'Confiding in crisis: gender differences in patterns of confiding among cancer patients', *Social Science & Medicine*, 41: 1255–60.

Haug, M. (1973) 'Deprofessionalisation: an alternative hypothesis for the future', *Sociological Review Monograph*, 20: 195–211.

Haug, M. (1988) 'A re-examination of the hypothesis of deprofessionalisation', *Milbank Quarterly*, 2(Supp.): 58–6.

Heidegger, M. (1927) *Sein und Zeit*, translated as *Being and Time* by John Macquarrie and Edward Robinson, Oxford: Basil Blackwell, 1978.

Henwood, F., Wyatt, S., Hart, A., and Smith, J. (2003) ' "Ignorance is bliss sometimes": constraints on the emergence of the "informed patient" in the changing landscapes of health information', *Sociology of Health & Illness*, 25(6): 589–607.

Hewson, M., Copeland, H., Mascha, E., Arrigain, S., Topol, E. and Fox, J. (2006) 'Integrative medicine: implementation and evaluation of a professional development program using experiential learning and conceptual change teaching approaches', *Patient Education and Counseling*, 62(1): 5–12.

Hirschkorn, K. and Bourgeault, I. (2005) 'Conceptualizing mainstream healthcare providers' behaviours in relation to complementary and alternative medicine', *Social Science & Medicine*, 61: 157–70.

House of Lords (2000) *Report on Complementary and Alternative Medicine*, London: House of Lords.

Ioannidis, J., Schmid, C. and Lau, J. (2000) 'Meta-analysis in hematology and oncology', *Hematology/Oncology Clinics of North America*, 14(4): 973–91.

Jacelon, C. and Imperio, K. (2005) 'Participant diaries as a source of data in research with older adults', *Qualitative Health Research*, 15(7): 991–7.

Jackson, S. and Scambler, G. (2007) 'Perceptions of evidence-based medicine: traditional acupuncturists in the UK and resistance to biomedical modes of evaluation', *Sociology of Health & Illness*, 29(3): 412–29.

Jarvis, W. (2005) 'How quackery harms cancer patients', *Quackwatch*; available online: http://www.quackwatch.org.

Jones, R. (2000) 'The unsolicited diary as a qualitative research tool for advanced research capacity in the field of health and illness', *Qualitative Health Research*, 10(4): 555–67.

Jordan, M. and Delunas, L. (2001) 'Quality of life and patterns of non-traditional therapy use by patients with cancer', *Oncology Nursing Forum*, 28(7): 1107–13.

Kakai, H., Maskarinec, G., Shumay, D., Tatsumura, T. and Tasaki, K. (2003) 'Ethnic differences in choices of health information by cancer patients using complementary and alternative medicine: an exploratory study with correspondence analysis', *Social Science & Medicine*, 56(4): 851–62.

Kaptchuk, T. and Eisenberg, D. (1998) 'The persuasive appeal of alternative medicine', *Annals of Internal Medicine*, 129(12): 1061–5.

Kelner, M., Wellman, B., Boon, H., and Welsh, S. (2004) 'Responses of established healthcare to the professionalization of complementary and alternative medicine in Ontario', *Social Science & Medicine*, 59: 915–30.

Kiley, R. (2002) 'Does the Internet harm health?', *British Medical Journal*, 324: 238.

Krizek, C., Roberts, C., Ragan, R., Ferrara, J. and Lord, B. (1999) 'Gender and cancer support group participation', *Cancer Practice*, 7(2): 86–92.

Lafferty, W., Bellas, A., Corage-Baden, A., Tyree, P., Standish, L. and Patterson, R. (2004) 'The use of complementary and alternative medical providers by insured cancer patients in Washington State', *Cancer*, 100(7): 1522–30.

Lambert, H. (2006) 'Accounting for EBM: notions of evidence in medicine', *Social Science & Medicine*, 62(11): 2633–45.

Larner, C. (1992) 'Healing in pre-industrial Britain', in Saks, M. (ed.) *Alternative Medicine in Britain*, Oxford: Clarendon Press.

Latour, B. (1987) *Science in Action: How to Follow Scientists and Engineers through Society*, Cambridge, MA: Harvard University Press.

Latour, B. (1988) *The Pasteurization of France*, Cambridge, MA: Harvard University Press.

Latour, B. (1993) *We Have Never Been Modern*, Cambridge, MA: Harvard University Press.

Latour, B. (1999) 'On recalling ANT', in Law, J. and Hassard, J. (eds) *Actor Network Theory and After*, Oxford: Blackwell Publishers.

Latour, B. (1999a) *Pandora's Hope: Essays on the Reality of Science Studies*, Cambridge, MA: Harvard University Press.

Latour, B. and Woolgar, S. (1979) *Laboratory Life: The Social Construction of Scientific Facts*, Beverly Hills: Sage Publications.

Law, J. (1992) 'Notes on the theory of actor network: ordering, strategy and heterogeneity', *Systems Practice*, 5(5): 379–94.

Law, J. (1994) *Organizing Modernity*, Oxford: Blackwell.

Law, J. (1999) 'After ANT: complexity, naming and topology', in Law, J. and Hassard, J. (eds) *Actor Network Theory and After*, Oxford: Blackwell Publishers.

Lea, J., Lockwood, G. and Ringash, J. (2005) 'Survey of computer use for health topics by patients with head and neck cancer', *Head and Neck*, 27(1): 8–14.

Lee, C. (2005) 'Communicating facts and knowledge in cancer complementary and alternative medicine', *Seminars in Oncology Nursing*, 21(3): 201–14.

Lee, M., Lin, S., Wrensch, M., Adler, S. and Eisenberg, D. (2000) 'Alternative therapies used by women with breast cancer in four ethnic populations', *Journal of the National Cancer Institute*, 92: 42–7.

Lee, M., Okazaki, S. and Yoo, H. (2006) 'Frequency and intensity of social anxiety in Asian Americans and European Americans', *Cultural Diversity and Ethnic Minority Psychology*, 12(2): 291–305.

Lengacher, C., Bennett, M., Kip, K., Gonzalez, L., Jacobsen, P. and Cox, C. (2006) 'Relief of symptoms, side effects, and psychological distress through use of complementary and alternative medicine in women with breast cancer', *Oncology Nursing Forum*, 33(1): 97–104.

Lewis, J., Marjoribanks, T. and Pirotta, M. (2003) 'Changing professions: general practitioners' perceptions of autonomy at the front line', *Journal of Sociology*, 39(1): 44–61.

Lewith, G., Broomfield, J. and Prescott, P. (2002) 'Complementary cancer care in Southampton', *Complementary Therapies in Medicine*, 10: 100–6.

Light, K. (1997) 'Florence Nightingale and holistic philosophy', *Journal of Holistic Nursing*, 15(1): 25–40.

Light, D. (2001) 'Managed competition, governmentality, and institutional response in the United Kingdom', *Social Science & Medicine*, 52: 1167–81.

Lofland, J. and Lofland, L. (1984) *Analyzing Social Settings: A Guide to Qualitative Observation and Analysis*, 2nd edition, Belmont, CA: Wadsworth.

Low, J. (2004) 'Managing safety and risk', *Health*, 8(4): 445–63.

Luff, D. and Thomas, K. (2000) 'Getting somewhere, feeling cared for: patient perspectives on CAM', *Complementary Therapies in Medicine*, 8: 253–59.

Lupton, D. (1995) *The Imperative of Health: Public Health and the Regulated Body*, London: Sage.

Lupton, D. (1997) 'Consumerism, reflexivity and the medical encounter', *Social Science & Medicine*, 45(3): 373–81.

Lupton, D. (1999) *Risk*, New York: Routledge.

Lupton, D. and Tulloch, J. (2002) ' "Risk is part of your life": risk epistemologies among a group of Australians', *Sociology*, 36(2): 317–35.

McClean, S. (2005) ' "The illness is part of the person": discourses of blame, individual responsibility and individuation at a centre for spiritual healing in the north of England', *Sociology of Health & Illness*, 27(5): 628–48.

Mackenzie, G., Parkinson, M., Lakhani, A. and Pannekoet, H. (1999) 'Issues that influence patient/physician discussion of complementary therapies', *Patient Education and Counselling*, 38: 155–9.

McKinley, J., Cattermole, H. and Oliver, C.W. (1999) 'The quality of surgical information on the Internet', *Journal of the Royal College of Surgeons of Edinburgh*, 44: 265–68.

Macleod, U., Ross, S., Gillis, C., McConnachie, A., Twelves, C. and Watt, G. (2000) 'Socioeconomic deprivation and stage of disease at presentation in women with breast cancer', *Annals of Oncology*, 11: 105–7.

Maly, R., Umezawa, Y., Ratliff, C. and Leake, B. (2006) 'Racial/ethnic group differences in treatment decision-making and treatment received among older breast carcinoma patients', *Cancer*, 106(4): 957–65.

Melton, J. (2001) *New Age Transformed*, Virginia: Institute for the Study of American Religion.

Mendelson, D. and Carino, T. (2005) 'Evidence-based medicine in the United States', *Health Affairs*, 24(1): 133–6.

Meth, P. (2003) 'Entries and omissions: using solicited diaries in geographical research', *Area*, 35(2): 195–205.

Metz, J., Devine, P. and DeNittis, A. (2003) 'A multi-institutional study of Internet utilization by radiation oncology patients', *International Journal of Radiation Oncology Biology Physics*, 56: 1201–5.

Milligan, M., Fanning, M., Hunter, S., Tadjali, M. and Stevens, E. (2002) 'Reflexology audit: patient satisfaction, impact on quality of life and availability in Scottish hospices', *International Journal of Palliative Nursing*, 8(10): 489–96.

Mizrachi, N., Shuval, J. and Gross, S. (2005) 'Boundary at work: alternative medicine in biomedical settings', *Sociology of Health & Illness*, 27(1): 20–43.

Molassiotis, A., Browall, M., Milovics, L., Panteli, V., Patiraki, E. and Fernandez-Ortega P. (2006) 'Complementary and alternative medicine use in patients with gynecological cancers in Europe', *International Journal of Gynaecological Cancer*, 16: 219–24.

Morris, K., Johnston, N., Homer, L. and Walts, D. (2000) 'A comparison of complementary therapy use between breast cancer patients and patients with other primary tumour sites', *American Journal of Surgery*, 179(5): 407–11.

Morrison, J., Sullivan, F., Murray, E. and Jolly, B. (1999) 'Evidence-based education', *Medical Education*, 33: 890–3.

Murdoch-Eaton, D. and Crombie, H. (2002) 'Complementary and alternative medicine in the undergraduate curriculum', *Medical Teacher*, 24(1): 100–3.

Murray, S. (2007) 'Care and the self: biotechnology, reproduction, and the good life', *Philosophy, Ethics, and Humanities in Medicine* 2(6); available online: http://www.peh-med.com/content/2/1/6.

Mykhalovskiy, E. (2003) 'Evidence-based medicine: ambivalent reading and the clinical recontextualization of science', *Health*, 7(3): 331–52.

Mykhalovskiy, E. and Weir, L. (2004) 'The problem of evidence-based medicine: directions for social science', *Social Science & Medicine*, 59(5): 1059–69.

NCCF (2003) Facts You Should Know about Childhood Cancer, Bethesda, MD: National Childhood Cancer Foundation.

NCI (1999) *Cancer Incidence and Survival among Children and Adolescents*: United States SEER Program 1975–1995, Bethesda, MD: National Cancer Institute.

Nettleton, S. and Burrows, R. (2003) 'E-scaped medicine?: Information, reflexivity and health', *Critical Social Policy*, 23(2): 165–85.

Nettleton, S., Burrows, R. and O'Malley, L. (2005) 'The mundane realities of the everyday lay use of the internet for health, and their consequences for media convergence', *Sociology of Health & Illness*, 27(7): 972–92.

ONS (2001) *Religion in Britain*, London: Office of National Statistics.

Passik, S. and Kirsh, K. (2000) 'The importance of quality-of-life endpoints in clinical trials to the practicing oncologist', *Hematology/Oncology Clinics of North America*, 14(4): 877–86.

Patterson, R., Neuhouser, M., Hedderson, M., Schwartz, S., Standish, L., Bowen, D. and Marshall, L. (2002) 'Types of alternative medicine used by patients with breast, colon, or prostate cancer: predictors, motives, and costs', *Journal Of Alternative and Complementary Medicine*, 8(4): 477–85.

Pham, B., Klassen, T., Lawson, M. and Moher, D. (2005) 'Language of publication restrictions in systematic reviews gave different results depending on whether the intervention was conventional or complementary', *Journal of Clinical Epidemiology* 58(8): 769–76.

Pittler, M.H. and Ernst, E. (2003) 'Systematic review: hepatotoxic events associated with herbal medicinal products', *Alimentary Pharmacology and Therapeutics*, 18(5): 451–71.

Pitts V. (2004) 'Illness and Internet empowerment: writing and reading breast cancer in cyberspace', *Health*, 8(1): 33–59.

Pope, C. (2003) 'Resisting evidence: the study of evidence-based medicine as a contemporary social movement', *Health*, 7(3): 267–82.

Quinn, M. and Babb, P. (2002) 'Patterns and trends in prostate cancer incidence, survival, prevalence and mortality. Part II: individual countries', *BJU International*, 90: 174–84.

Quinn, M., Babb, P., Brock, A., Kirby, E. and Jones, J. (2001) *Cancer Trends in England and Wales 1950–1999*, Studies on Medical and Population Subject No. 66. London: The Stationery Office.

Radin, P. (2006) ' "To me, it's my life": medical communication, trust, and activism in cyberspace', *Social Science & Medicine*, 62: 591–601.

Ramsey, S.D., Berry, K., Moinpour, C., Giedzinska, A. and Andersen, M. (2002) 'Quality of life in long term survivors of colorectal cancer', *American Journal of Gastroenterology*, 97: 1228–34.

Rayner, L. and Easthope, G. (2001) 'Postmodern consumption and alternative medications', *Journal of Sociology*, 37(2): 157–76.

Rees, R., Feigel, I., Vickers, A., Zollman, C., McGurk, R. and Smith, C. (2000) 'Prevalence of complementary therapy use by women with breast cancer', *European Journal of Cancer*, 36: 1359–64.

Richardson, M.A., Sanders, T., Palmer, J.L., Greisinger, A. and Singletary, S.E. (2000) 'Complementary/alternative medicine use in a comprehensive cancer center and the implications for oncology', *Journal of Clinical Oncology*, 18: 2505–14.

Roberts, C., Baker, F., Hann, D., Runfola, J., Witt, C., McDonald, J., Livingston, M., Ruiterman, J., Ampela, R., Kaw, O. and Blanchard, C. (2005) 'Patient–physician communication regarding use of complementary therapies during cancer treatment', *Journal of Psychosocial Oncology*, 23(4): 35–60.

Ross, C., Hamilton, J., Macrae, G., Docherty, C., Gould, A. and Cornbleet, M. (2002) 'A pilot study to evaluate the effect of reflexology on mood and symptom rating of advanced cancer patients', *Palliative Medicine*, 16: 544–5.

Rose, N. (1999) *Governing the Soul*, 2nd edition, London: Free Association Books.

Rose, N. (2001) 'The politics of life itself', *Theory, Culture and Society*, 18(6): 1–30.

Rubin, H. and Rubin, I. (1995) *Qualitative Interviewing: The Art of Hearing Data*, London: Sage.

Sackett, D., Straus, S., Richardson, S., Rosenberg, W. and Haynes, R. (2000) 'Evidence-based medicine: how to practice and teach EBM, 2nd edition, London: Churchill Livingstone.

Saks, M. (ed.) (1992) *Alternative Medicine in Britain*, Oxford: Clarendon Press.

Saks, M. (1994) 'The alternatives to medicine', in Gabe, J., Kelleher, D. and Williams, G. (eds) *Challenging Medicine*, London: Routledge.

Saks, M. (1995) *Professions and the Public Interest: Medical Power, Altruism and Alternative Medicine*, London: Routledge.

Saks, M. (1996) 'From quackery to complementary medicine: the shifting boundaries between orthodox and unorthodox medical knowledge', in Cant, S. and Sharma, U. (eds) *Complementary and Alternative Medicines: Knowledge in Practice*, London: Free Association Books.

Saks, M. (1998) 'Medicine and complementary medicine: challenge and change', in Scambler, G. and Higgs, P. (eds) *Modernity Medicine and Health*, London: Routledge.

Samson, C. (1999) 'Biomedicine and the body', in Samson, C. (ed.) *Health Studies: A Critical and Cross-Cultural Reader*, Oxford: Blackwell Publishers.

Schmidt, K. and Ernst, E. (2004) 'Assessing websites on complementary and alternative medicine for cancer', *Annals of Oncology*, 15(5): 733–42.

Scott, A. (1998) 'Homoeopathy as a feminist form of medicine', *Sociology of Health & Illness* 20(2): 191–215.

Scott, J., Kearney, N., Hummerston, S. and Molassiotis, A. (2005) 'Use of complementary and alternative medicine in patients with cancer: a UK survey', *European Journal of Oncology Nursing*, 29(2): 131–7.

Seale, C. (2005) 'New directions for critical internet health studies: representing cancer experience on the web', *Sociology of Health & Illness*, 27(4): 515–40.

Seale, C., Ziebland, S. and Charteris-Black, J. (2006) 'Gender, cancer experience and internet use: a comparative keyword analysis of interviews and online cancer support groups', *Social Science and Medicine*, 62(10): 2577–90.

Sharf, B. (1997) 'Communicating breast cancer on-line: support and empowerment on the Internet', *Women and Health*, 26(1): 65–84.

Siahpush, M. (1998) 'Postmodern values, dissatisfaction with conventional medicine and popularity of alternative therapies', *Journal of Sociology*, 34(1): 58–70.

Sirois, F. and Gick, M. (2002) 'An investigation of the health beliefs and motivations of complementary medicine clients', *Social Science & Medicine* 55(6): 1025–37.

Smith, B. (1999) 'Ethical and methodological benefits of using a reflexive journal in hermeneutic phenomenologic research', *Image: Journal of Nursing Scholarship*, 31(4): 359–63.

Soden, K., Vincent, K., Craske, S., Lucas, Surrey, E. and Ashley, S. (2004) 'A randomized controlled trial of aromatherapy massage in a hospice setting', *Palliative Medicine*, 18: 87–92.

Sointu, E. (2006) 'The search for wellbeing in alternative and complementary health practices', *Sociology of Health & Illness*, 28(3): 330–49.

Star, S.L. and Griesemer, J.R. (1989) 'Institutional ecology, "translations" and boundary objects', *Social Studies of Science*, 19: 387–420.

Stead, M., Fallowfield, L., Brown, J. and Selby, P. (2001) 'Communication about sexual problems and sexual concerns in ovarian cancer: qualitative study', *British Medical Journal*, 323(7317): 836–7.

Stephenson, N., Weinrich, S. and Tavakoli, A. (2000) 'The effects of foot reflexology on anxiety and pain in patients with breast and lung cancer', *Oncology Nursing Forum*, 27: 67–72.

Stoll, C. (1995) *Silicon Snake Oil*, New York: Doubleday.

Strauss, A. and Corbin, J. (1990) *Basics of Qualitative Research: Grounded Theory Procedures and Techniques*, Newbury Park, CA: Sage Publications.

Tasaki, K., Maskarinec, G., Shumay, D., Tatsumura, Y. and Kakai, H. (2002) 'Communication between physicians and cancer patients about complementary and alternative medicine: exploring patients' perspectives', *Psycho-Oncology*, 11: 212–20.

Tavares, M. (2003) *National Guidelines for the Use of Complementary Therapies in Supportive and Palliative Care*, United Kingdom: The Prince of Wales' Foundation for Integrated Health.

Thomas, K., Nicholl, J. and Coleman, P. (2001) 'Use and expenditure on complementary medicine in England', *Complementary Therapies in Medicine*, 9: 2–11.

Timmermans, S. and Kolker, E. (2004) 'Evidence-based medicine and the reconfiguration of medical knowledge', *Journal of Health and Social Behavior*, 45 (extra issue): 177–93.

Tovey, P. (2003) 'Group mediation of complementary and alternative medicine in cancer care in the UK and Pakistan', *European Journal of Cancer Care*, 12: 374–5.

Tovey, P. and Adams, J. (2001) 'Primary care as intersecting social worlds', *Social Science & Medicine*, 52: 695–706.

Tovey, P. and Adams, J. (2002) 'Towards a sociology of CAM and nursing', *Complementary Therapies in Nursing and Midwifery*, 8: 12–16.

Tovey, P. and Adams, J. (2003) 'Nostalgic and nostophobic referencing and the authentication of nurses' use of complementary therapies', *Social Science and Medicine*, 56: 1469–80.

Tovey, P. and Broom, A. (2007) 'Cancer patients' negotiation of therapeutic options in Pakistan', *Qualitative Health Research*, 17(5): 652–62.

Tovey, P. and Broom, A. (2007a) 'Oncologists' and specialist cancer nurses' approaches to complementary and alternative medicine use and their impact on patient action', *Social Science and Medicine*, 64: 2550–64.

Tovey, P., Atkin, K. and Milewa, T. (2001) 'The individual and primary care: service user, reflexive choice maker and collective actor', *Critical Public Health*, 11(2): 153–66.

Tovey, P., Chatwin, J. and Broom, A. (2007) *Traditional, Complementary and Alternative Medicine and Cancer Care: An International Analysis of Grassroots Integration*, Routledge: London and New York.

Tredaniel, J., Blay, J., Goldwasser, F., Asselain, B., Koscielny, S., de Labareyre, C., Balogh, N., Bismut, H., Misset, J. and Marty M. (2005) 'Decision-making process in oncology practice: is the information available and what should it consist of?', *Critical Reviews in Oncology-Hematology*, 54(3): 165–70.

Tudiver, F. and Talbot, Y. (1999) 'Why men don't seek help? Family physicians' perspectives on health-seeking behaviour in men', *Journal of Family Practice*, 43: 475–80.

Turner, B.S. and Samson, C. (1995) *Medical Power and Social Knowledge*, 2nd edition, London: Sage Publications.

Turner, J., Zapart, S., Pedersen, K., Rankin, N., Luxford, K. and Fletcher, J. (2005) 'Clinical practice guidelines for the psychosocial care of adults with cancer', *Psycho-Oncology*, 14: 159–73.

Vickers, A. (2000) 'Recent advances: complementary medicine', *British Medical Journal*, 321: 683–6.

Vigna-Taglianti, F., Vineis, P., Liberati, A. and Faggiano, F. (2006) 'Quality of systematic reviews used in guidelines for oncology practice', *Annals of Oncology*, 17(4): 691–701.

Villanueva-Russell, Y. (2005) 'Evidence-based medicine and its implications for the profession of chiropractic', *Social Science and Medicine*, 60: 545–61.

Vincent, S. and Djulbegovic, B. (2005) 'Oncology treatment recommendations can be supported only by 1–2% of high-quality published evidence', *Cancer Treatment Review*, 31(4): 319–22.

Von Gruenigen, V.E., White, L.J., Kirven, M.S., Showalter, A.L., Hopkins, M.P. and Jenison, E.L. (2001) 'A comparison of complementary and alternative medicine use by gynecology and gynecologic oncology patients', *International Journal of Gynecological Cancer*, 11(3): 205–9.

Waddington, I. (1973) 'The struggle to reform the Royal College of Physicians 1767–1771: a sociological analysis', *Medical History*, 17: 107–26.

Wainwright, D. (1997) 'Can sociological research be qualitative, critical and valid?', *The Qualitative Report*, 3(2); available online: http://www.nova.edu/sss/QR/QRs–2/wain.html.

Weiger, W., Smith, M., Boon, H., Richardson, M., Kaptchuk, T. and Eisenberg, D. (2002) 'Advising patients who seek complementary and alternative medical therapies for cancer', *Annals of Internal Medicine*, 137: 889–903.

White, A., Resch, K. and Ernst, E. (1997) 'Complementary medicine: use and attitudes among general practitioners', *Family Practice*, 14: 302–6.

White, R. (2002) 'Social and political aspects of men's health', *Health*, 6(3): 267–85.

Whiting, R. (2000). 'A healthy way to learn: the medical community assesses online health-care', *Information Week*; available online: http://www.informationweek.com/816/kin4.htm (accessed 10 June 2007).

Wilkinson, Jenny M. and Simpson, Maree D. (2001) 'High use of complementary therapies in a New South Wales rural community', *Australian Journal of Rural Health*, 9(4), August: 166–171.

Willis, E. (1989) *Medical Dominance: The Division of Labour in Australian Health Care*, Sydney: Allen and Unwin.

Willis, E. (1994) *Illness and Social Relations: Issues in the Sociology of Health Care*, St Leonards, NSW: Allen and Unwin.

Willis, E. (2003) 'The politics of evidence and the evidence for CAM', *Healthcare Papers*, 5(3): 37–42.

Willis, E. (2006) 'Introduction: taking stock of medical dominance', *Health Sociology Review*, 15(2): 1–12.

Willis, E. and Coulter, Ian (2004) 'The rise and rise of complementary and alternative medicine: a sociological perspective', *Medical Journal of Australia*, 180(11): 587–9.

Willis, E. and White, K. (2002) 'Positivism resurgent: the epistemological foundations of evidence-based medicine', *Health Sociology Review*, 11(2): 5–15.

Wilson, K. and Mills, E. (2002) 'Evidence-based complementary and alternative medicine working group', *Journal of Alternative and Complementary Medicine*, 8(2): 103–5.

Wray, S. (2007) 'Health, exercise and wellbeing: the experiences of midlife women from diverse ethnic backgrounds', *Social Theory & Health*, 5(2): 126–45.

Wright, P., Smith, A., Booth, L., Winterbottom, A., Kiely, M., Velikova, G. and Selby, P. (2005) 'Psychosocial difficulties, deprivation and cancer: three questionnaire studies involving 609 cancer patients', *British Journal of Cancer*, 93: 622–6.

Ziebland, S. (2004) 'The importance of being expert: the quest for cancer information on the Internet', *Social Science & Medicine*, 59: 1783–93.

Ziebland, S., Chapple, A., Dumelow, C., Evans, J., Prinjha, S. and Rozmovits, L. (2004) 'How the internet affects patients' experience of cancer: a qualitative study', *British Medical Journal*, 328: 564.

Zimmerman, D.H., and Wieder, D.L. (1977) 'The diary interview method', *Urban Life*, 5(4): 479–99.

Zollman, C. and Vickers, A. (1999) 'Complementary medicine and the doctor – ABC of complementary medicine', *British Medical Journal*, 319: 1558–61.

Index